THE
Aromatherapy
AND *Massage*
BOOK

IMPORTANT

Although essential oils are used by French doctors in the treatment of serious illnesses, with oral doses of the oils playing a major role, it is important to point out here that it would be far too ambitious (and potentially risky) for the lay person and, indeed, the average aromatherapist, to attempt treating chronic illness wih essential oils, whether applied externally or taken by mouth. Aromatherapy, as it is more usually practised, is about the *prevention* of major illness through the medium of massage, enhanced by the physiological and psycho-therapeutic effects of plant essences.

* **Never take essential oils internally**
* **Never use an essential oil about which you can find little or no information**
* **During pregnancy, whilst breastfeeding, and for children under twelve years old, it is advisable to use oils in half the stated quantities**
* **Never use essential oils for babies or young children, except under the guidance of a qualified aromatherapist.**

Thorsons
An Imprint of HarperCollins*Publishers*
77–85 Fulham Palace Road
Hammersmith, London W6 8JB

Published by Thorsons 1994
10 9 8 7 6 5 4 3 2

A CIP catalogue record for this book is available from the British Library

ISBN 0 7225 29759

Design: Bev Speight
Editorial: Liz Dean
Cover photography: Monique Le Luhandre
Massage photography: Sue Atkinson
Picture Research: Bev Speight & Liz Dean
Illustration: Claire Hedges
Lettering: Nigel Wright
Models: Robin, Juliet Seatree & Lauren, Bev Speight

Picture Credits: Art Directors Photo Library, David Armstrong, The Bridgeman Art Library, Sue Atkinson, Telegraph Colour Library UK, The C.W. Daniel Co Ltd, photo of Gattefossé from *Gattefossé's Aromatherapy*, ICOREC, The *International Journal of Aromatherapy*.

Produced by HarperCollins Hong Kong

Contents

To Rose, with love.

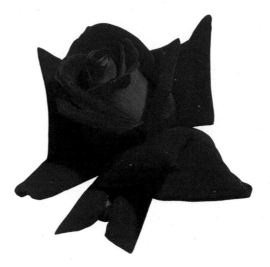

Acknowledgements
*Many thanks to Jane Graham Maw for suggesting this project
in the first place – and to everyone else at Thorsons for their
hard work and dedication. I am especially grateful to Liz Dean
for her meticulous editorial eye, and for her encouragement
and support. I would also like to thank Sue Atkinson for the
excellent photography, and Beverley Speight for the beautiful
and imaginative design work – it's a joy to behold!*

THE Aromatherapy AND Massage BOOK

CHRISTINE WILDWOOD

Thorsons
An Imprint of HarperCollins*Publishers*

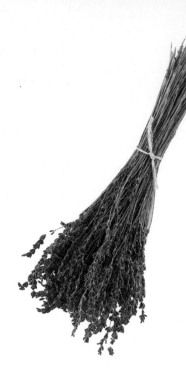

Introduction

The beautiful ancient art of aromatherapy combines the healing properties of aromatic plant essences – or essential oils – with massage, thus making good use of our sense of smell and touch. Add gentle music and a pleasing decor, and we also heighten our sense of hearing and sight. Blend some mood-enhancing aromas and apply with tender loving care, and we are nurtured physically, emotionally and mentally.

Essential oils can be used in a variety of ways for healing or simply for pleasure. They can be blended into vegetable oils and creams for skin care, added to the bath, used in steam inhalations for colds and influenza, blended into enchanting perfumes, vaporized to create an enjoyable ambience in the home, and much more besides.

Aromatherapy massage, however, is the mainstay of the art and therefore the focus of this book. Included is a full-body massage routine accompanied by illustrated step-by-step sequences, with advice on massaging babies, children and elderly people, plus plenty of ideas for some wonderful aromatic blends.

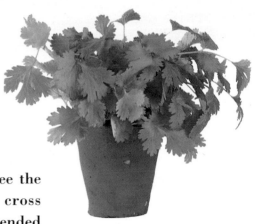

To find out about the therapeutic properties of essential oils, see the thirty essential oil profiles in Chapter 3, and the therapeutic cross reference chart in Chapter 7, which displays a list of oils recommended for the symptomatic treatment of minor ailments.

Aromatherapy is particularly helpful for soothing the detrimental effects of stress. Stress, in its many guises, accounts for the vast majority of ills in this world of speed, 'high tec' and emotional unrest. However, it is important to bear in mind that aromatherapy, like other holistic therapies, works best when it is incorporated with a healthy diet and lifestyle. By aiming to stimulate rather than suppress the body's natural defences, aromatherapy helps create favourable conditions in both body and mind for our self-healing ability to come to the fore.

However, you need not be ill to benefit from essential oils. As you are about to discover in the following pages, aromatherapy is a natural and pleasurable way to find tranquillity, restore vitality and to enhance our aesthetic sense of harmony.

Chrisse Wildwood

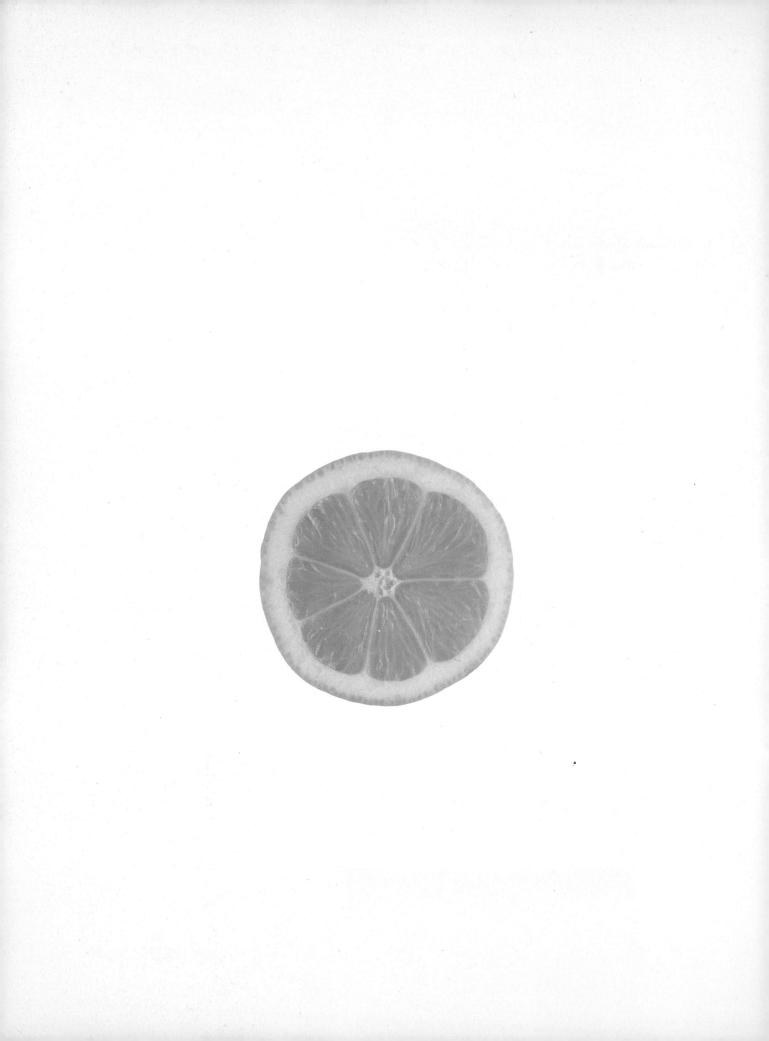

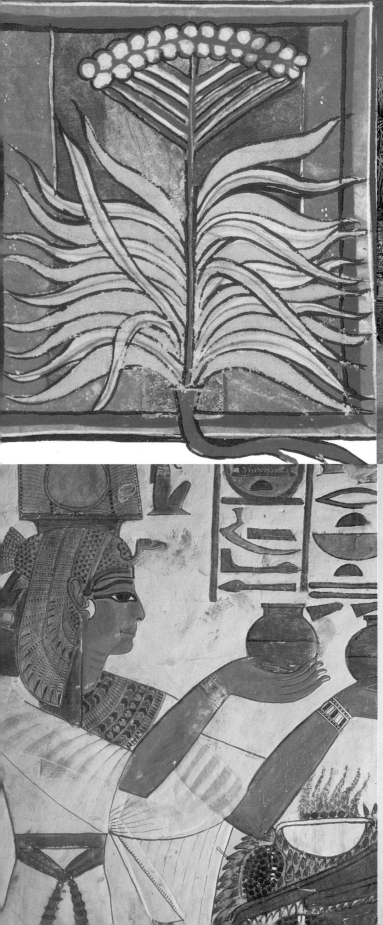
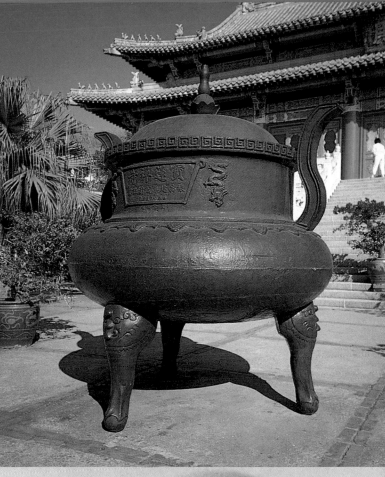

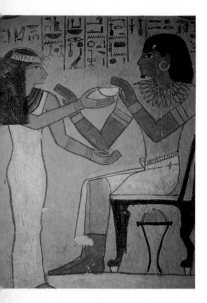

People have always been enchanted by the seemingly magical powers of aromatic plants. Thousands of years ago, our early ancestors used their highly developed senses and intuition to find out which plants were edible and able to be used for healing and which were poisonous. Most fascinating of all were those that could induce altered states of consciousness. It was discovered that when certain aromatic plants and plant resins were burnt as incense, some fragrances made people feel relaxed or drowsy while others made them feel ecstatic or euphoric. The most prized plants of all were those burned by priests and priestesses during religious rites to cure the sick, and those which were believed to conjure up mystical experiences.

Until the growth of mainstream western medicine in the eighteenth century, healing and religious practice were always closely connected. The 'smoking' of sick people was a common element of the healer's art and involved burning plants to exorcise evil spirits. We still use words associated with that today – the word perfume is derived from the Latin for 'through the smoke'.

Ancient Egypt

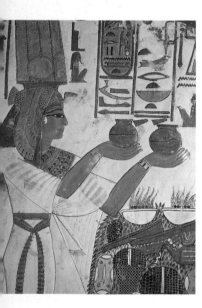

The true founders of aromatherapy were the ancient Egyptians. They used aromatics in rituals and healing, including different forms of massage, and for cosmetics and embalming. The survival of mummies bears witness not just to the embalmers' skills, but to the extraordinary preservative powers of the plant essences they used. When Tut'ankhamun's tomb was opened in 1922, archaeologists discovered a pot of ointment that had retained its fragrance. More recently when a 3,000-year-old mummy was unwrapped, the aromas of myrrh and cedarwood could be detected on the inner bandages.

The formulae for many aromatic concoctions were carved into the stone walls of Egyptian temples so, today, we can still enjoy the fruits of their astounding preparations. Sixteen ingredients including saffron, cassia, spikenard, cinnamon and juniper went to make up kyphi, the forerunner of the perfume base known today as chypre. The Ancient Egyptians always burned it after sunset, not only to ensure the safe return of the Sun God Ra, but also because its effects were soporific and intoxicating. Theriaque, another complex cocktail, thought to dispel anxiety, had anything between fifty-seven and ninety-six components – temple recipes vary – but myrrh, cinnamon, rush, sweet flag, juniper and cassia were regularly used – often with a less aesthetic seasoning of serpent skin, crocodile dung and spittle!

Ancient China

China, too, has always had a long and respectable aromatherapy tradition. In ancient times, wealthy Chinese households reserved a special room for childbirth where the plant mugwort (*Artemisia vulgaris*) was burned to help labour and was believed to be soothing for the newborn infant. A quest for immortality haunted the ancient Chinese, who used alchemy in a bid to discover its secret. An alchemist would ceremoniously burn incense and douse himself with specially prepared perfume before carrying out his experiments. The belief was that the plants' fragrance acted as a vehicle for magical forces and spirits which would unveil the mysteries of eternal life.

The Magic of Frankincense

Throughout the ancient world frankincense resin, extracted from trees grown in south-west Arabia, was traded. Its highly regarded spiritual properties gave it a higher value than gold. People believed deeply that when frankincense was burned, its aromatic vapour sent the human spirit soaring to meet the sublime energy of the gods. Frankincense gave humanity a glimpse of the divine.

Modern science offers a partial vindication. In 1981 German scientists decided to investigate the so-called mind-bending effects of inhaling the aroma of frankincense, which is still burned in Catholic churches. Altar boys were said to have become emotionally addicted to it. Analysis revealed that when burned, vapours from the substance contain a psychoactive chemical which stimulates the subconscious.

Scientific Advance

It was Arab physicians who instinctively harnessed the powerful germicidal properties of essential oils by disinfecting their bodies and clothes with sandalwood, camphor and rosewater. This practice was also encouraged by Hippocrates as a way of warding off infection.

The eleventh-century Arab, Avicenna, gave aromatherapy a lasting practical scientific application. To capture the ethereal plant essences, he perfected a process, begun in Mesopotamia, known as distillation. So advanced were Avicenna's methods that the apparatus for distillation has barely altered in 900 years (see page 17).

The wonders of Arabian perfumes spread beyond the Ancient world to Europe, brought back by knights returning from the Crusades. While the ancients of the Middle and Far East were as concerned about cleanliness as modern societies, malodorous medieval Europe lagged

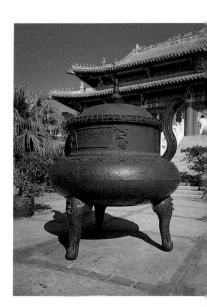

Tripod for burning incense – outside Buddhist temple, Hong Kong

behind. However, the crusading knights changed all this because, along with the perfumes, they also brought back the knowledge of how to distil them.

The Normans, too, had a hand in bringing aromatherapy to Britain. One especially therapeutic custom was to spread sweet-smelling plants on the floor which gave off pervasive scents when crushed underfoot. Many had insecticidal and bactericidal properties which helped counter airborne infection and deterred lice and fleas.

New perfumes and ideas encouraged people to smother their unwashed bodies and clothes with fragrances. It became fashionable to carry around little bouquets of aromatic herbs, known as tussie mussies, to ward off illness and to mask the stench of the streets.

Gradually it became evident that when plague struck, perfumers, who were pervaded with essential oils, remained immune. This led to the development of the famous Four Thieves' Vinegar, a potion so called because a quartet of robbers in Marseille during the Great Plague in 1722 would rub themselves all over with it before plundering the bodies of stricken victims. The ingredients of this remarkable mixture included a concentration of garlic along with the essences of rosemary, camphor, lavender, nutmeg, sage and cinnamon, suspended in vinegar.

By the seventeenth century the emergence of synthetic and chemical drugs sidelined the use of herbs and essential oils in medicine. Mercury, for example, proved especially popular for the treatment of syphilis. In her book *Green Pharmacy*, Barbara Griggs describes the horrific side-effects of this treatment: disintegration of the jaw, tremors and occasionally even total paralysis. Although in some cases the syphilis was eradicated, the treatment certainly killed great numbers of patients. In retrospect, dying of the disease itself would seem infinitely preferable to the agonies of death from mercury poisoning.

It was in the nineteenth century, however, that a pattern was established that continues today; chemists were intent on sifting out the so-called impurities of plants in order to isolate their 'active principles'. However, what were regarded as impurities are often a necessary constituent because they work in harmony with the active principle, thus reducing the possibility of side effects. Nevertheless, it is important to stress that not all substances occurring in nature are benign. Take laurel leaves, from which cyanide is derived, and the foxglove which contains the cardiac tranquilliser digitalis – both in quantity can be lethal.

Twentieth-century Pioneers

Rene-Maurice Gattefossé

It was Gattefossé, the French cosmetic scientist, who coined the term 'aromatherapy' in 1937 when he used it as the title for his book on the subject. At first his research was confined to the cosmetic uses of essential oils, but he soon realized that many oils also had powerful antiseptic properties. The most remarkable instance of this was when Gattefossé was badly burned in a laboratory explosion. He treated the wound with lavender essence, which helped it heal so completely that not even a scar was left.

Following Gattefossé's research into the properties of essential oils, a great deal of interest was generated in France and Italy. Not only were the oils found to heal skin and strengthen immunity, they were also capable of relieving mental conditions such as anxiety and depression.

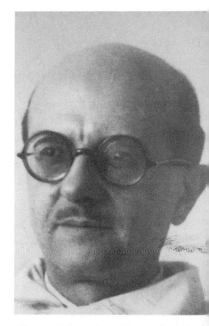

Rene-Maurice Gattefossé

Paolo Rovesti

Professor Paolo Rovesti of Milan demonstrated that smelling oils of certain plants induced a feeling of optimism. Taking oils from local products like bergamot, orange and lemon, he soaked bits of cotton wool in essential oils and passed them under the noses of his patients who were then said to undergo a profound release of pent-up emotions.

Jean Valnet

The French physician Dr Jean Valnet, an ex-army surgeon, contributed most to the medical assessment and acceptance of aromatherapy.

Valnet used essential oils to treat the wounds of soldiers during the Second World War. Later, in his book *Aromatherapie*, he describes how he successfully treated several long-term psychiatric patients with essential oils. These people were also suffering physical side-effects from the drugs administered to them for control of depression and hallucinations. Valnet's treatment involved weaning them off the drugs, and using essential oils in conjunction with a special diet. He reported distinct improvements in all symptoms, sometimes within days of starting the therapy. His book, *The Practice of Aromatherapy*, has become a classic for practitioners.

Marguerite Maury

The Austrian-born biochemist Marguerite Maury has been hailed as the mother of holistic aromatherapy. Although inspired by Gattefossé, she developed a special massage technique which involved applying essential oils along the nerve centres of the spine, believing that they worked more profoundly when inhaled or absorbed by the skin rather than taken orally.

She also introduced the idea of the individual prescription whereby oils were chosen according to the individual needs of her clients. The clients, mainly wealthy women seeking rejuvenation, reported dramatic improvement in their skin's condition, along with some surprising side-effects. Many experienced relief from rheumatic pain, slept more deeply and enjoyed a generally improved mental state. The effects lasted weeks, sometimes months, after the end of treatment.

Marguerite Maury was totally dedicated to her work and, in 1962 and 1967, was rewarded with two international prizes for her research. Soon after, aged seventy-three, she died of a stroke, thought to be due to overwork.

Her achievements are best described by her husband and colleague, the homoeopathic physician Dr E.A. Maury, who says: 'She continues to show the way for those who have been willing to recognize her and will long do so for those who seek a new way of achieving moral and physical well being'.

Robert Tisserand

Robert Tisserand, a British aromatherapist, author and researcher, has arguably generated the most popular interest in aromatherapy. In his book *The Art of Aromatherapy* (1977), he discusses the history, therapeutic properties and applications of a number of essential oils. The work has become a bestseller in its field.

Tisserand also helped to found two aromatherapy associations and is the editor of the *International Journal of Aromatherapy*.

Popular Awareness

The increasing number of books on aromatherapy, a great deal of media attention and its recent introduction into National Health Service hospitals, all demonstrate the enormous leap that aromatherapy has made from relative obscurity into the spotlight of popular awareness.

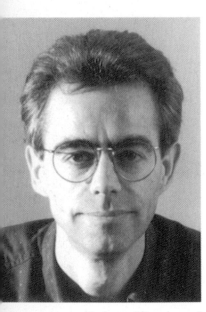

Robert Tisserand

What makes it so special? ... Read on.

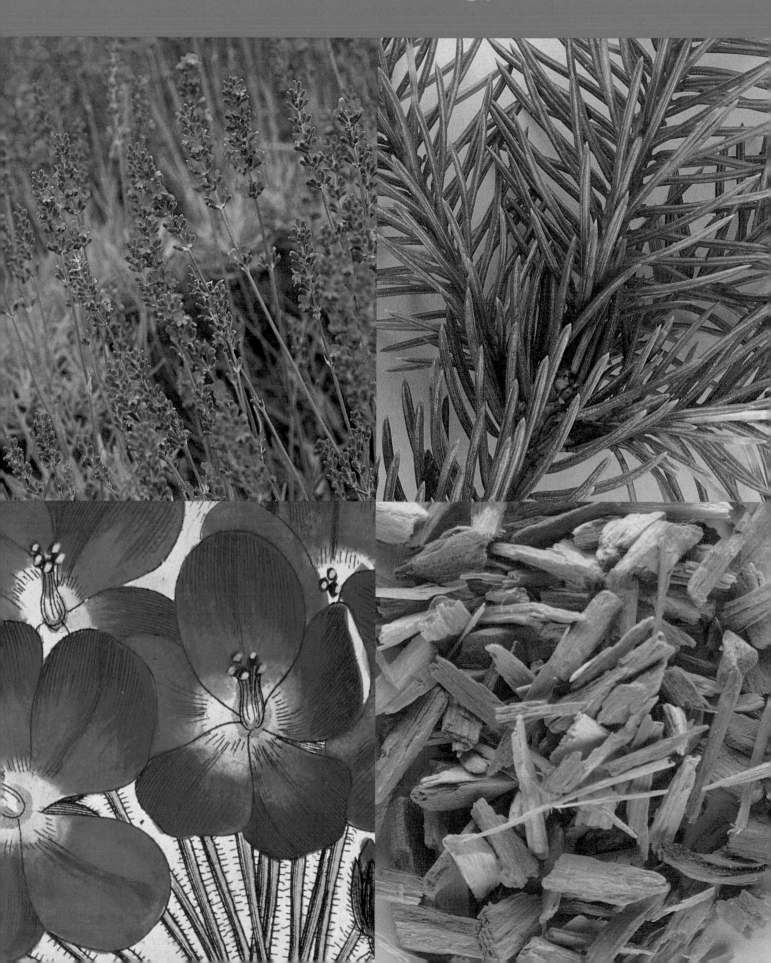

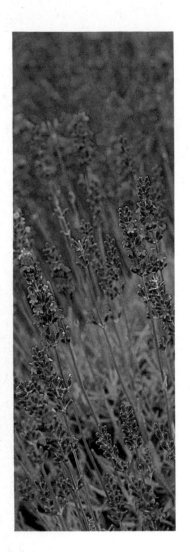

Aromatherapy works in two interrelated ways. First there is the aroma of the oil and its effect on the emotions; secondly, there is the pharmacological action of the oil and its effect on the bodily systems. As a bonus, when the aromatherapy massage is performed with sensitivity, an empathy develops between the giver and the receiver, and the treatment becomes a powerful form of hands-on-healing.

To understand better how aromatherapy works, we need to look more closely at the essential oils and see how they interact to benefit body and mind.

What are Essential Oils?

Essential oils are the fragrant liquid components of aromatic plants, trees and grasses. They are sometimes called 'ethereal oils', a Germanic term which sums up their elusive nature – if they are left in the open air they quickly evaporate.

The oils are contained in tiny oil glands or sacs which are concentrated in different parts of the plant. They may be found in the petals (rose), the leaves (eucalyptus), the roots of grass (vetiver), the heart, or soft wood found under the bark (sandalwood), the fruit (lemon), the seeds (caraway), the rhizomes (ginger), the resin (pine). Sometimes the oil is yielded from more than one part of the plant. For instance, lavender yields oil from both its flowers and leaves; and the versatile orange tree produces three different essences, each with a specific therapeutic property: the heady bitter-sweet neroli (flowers), the similar, though less refined scent of petitgrain (leaves) and the outer orange scent (skin of the fruit).

The more oil glands or sacs present in the plant, the cheaper the oil is to buy and vice versa. A hundred kilos of lavender yields almost three litres of essential oil, whereas one hundred kilos of rose petals produces only a half-litre of oil. Although some essential oils are very expensive, especially rose otto and neroli oils, they are highly concentrated substances and, if used correctly, as explained in this book, will last a long time.

Although essential oils may be technically classified as oils, they are, in fact, quite different from ordinary 'fixed oils' such as corn or sunflower. They are highly volatile (easily vaporized) and do not leave a permanent mark on paper. Unlike fatty vegetable oils, most essential oils have a consistency closer to water or alcohol and are not at all greasy. However, some are viscous (vetiver, myrrh) and rose otto is semi-solid at low temperatures. Essential oils are also soluble in wax, such as melted beeswax or jojoba, egg yolk, alcohol and vegetable oils. Even though they are not entirely water soluble, they are successful as bath oils or for use in skin and hair tonics if the water is agitated to disperse the fine droplets.

How are Essential Oils Extracted?

The classic method is by steam distillation. This is a sophisticated version of an ancient method that was first devised in Mesopotamia over 5,000 years ago. Plant material is piled into a still and subjected to concentrated steam, which releases the essential oils from the plant cells. The aromatic vapour is then sent on its travels along a series of glass tubes which act as a condenser, and the oil is separated from the water when siphoned through a narrow-necked container. The remaining water may form a fragrant by-product: for example, rosewater, orange flower water and lavender water.

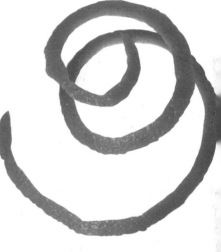

The essences of citrus fruits such as orange, lemon, bergamot and mandarin, are found in the rind and are obtained by a simple process known as expression. Although this was once carried out by hand – by squeezing the rind – machines using centrifugal force have now replaced this technique.

Enfleurage was a once-common means of extraction. This entails using animal fat, usually lard, to absorb the essences, which are then separated out using alcohol. The evaporation of the alcohol leaves the essential oil. *Enfleurage* is still used by some perfumers to capture the fragrances of flowers such as jasmine, orange flower and tuberose whose delicate aromas can be spoiled by the intense heat of distillation. If you can actually find such an extraction, it will be labelled 'enfleurage absolute', not 'essential oil', and will be very expensive. Only a few *enfleurage absolutes* reach suppliers.

The high cost involved in this labour-intensive and time-consuming *enfleurage* method has led to the wide use of solvents such as hexane and petroleum ether, plus the occasional use of benzene, a carcinogenic substance. Quite apart from concern about the traces of solvent left behind in absolutes, there is also concern about these substances being discharged into the atmosphere. Although the extraction process itself is carried out in sealed containers and the solvent recycled, the discarded solvent-saturated plant matter is thrown on the rubbish heap and can be a pollutant. These solvent-produced oils are widely available from essential oil suppliers and are labelled 'absolute'. With the exception of rose otto, they are more expensive than most essential oils, but are not as costly as the *enfleurage absolutes*.

The most recent method of extraction uses low-temperature carbon dioxide which produces some exquisite aromas. Although an expensive process, it is ideal for people who are unhappy about solvent extraction. Certainly carbon dioxide extraction is thought to be a cleaner alternative to potentially toxic solvents. The only drawback, apart from cost, is availability. Few essential oil suppliers stock these oils. If you do find them, they will be labelled 'CO_2'.

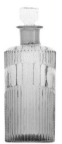

What are Organically Produced Oils?

Organically produced oils are those extracted from plants grown without the use of chemical fertilizers and sprays. Unfortunately not all oils are organically produced. Oils that are labelled 'organic' tend to be derived from herbs – for example, lavender, rosemary, marjoram and camomile. Some oils, however, particularly frankincense and those extracted from other disease-resistant trees such as cypress, pine and myrrh come from unsprayed crops. Other essential oils such as ylang-ylang and sandalwood, are imported from countries where chemical sprays and fertilizers are not in general use.

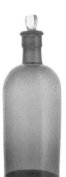

Of course, all essential oils are organic in the sense that they are extracted from living plants. To avoid being misled, always purchase from well-respected suppliers (see Appendix). For instance, you may be charged extra for an 'organic' ylang-ylang essence when, in reality, practically all the world's supply of ylang-ylang is produced using non-toxic methods of cultivation. However, you may come across an exorbitantly priced bottle of 'organic' rose or jasmine – expensive oils in any case – when almost all rose and jasmine plantations are regularly sprayed and fertilized by laboratory produced chemicals.

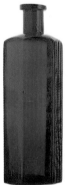

If you wish to use only environmentally-friendly products, avoid rosewood oil, also known as Bois de Rose. This is extracted from trees torn down in the threatened rainforests of South America and Africa.

What are the Properties of Essential Oils?

Essential oils are an aromatic plant's survival kit. They serve many purposes – they influence growth and reproduction, attract pollinating insects, repel predators and ward off disease. It is a survival kit that can work well for people, too. For example, studies have shown that the essential oils of lavender and neroli promote the growth of healthy skin cells. Others, such as fennel, rose and cypress, influence

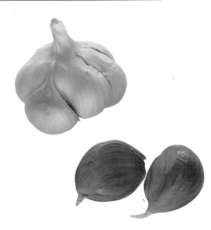

hormonal secretions, thus benefiting the reproductive system. Many oils, notably rosemary, geranium and eucalyptus kill head lice, and oils such as tea tree, garlic and thyme actually help to strengthen the immune system.

As for 'attracting pollinating insects', essential oils such as sandalwood, rose otto, ylang-ylang and patchouli have been credited with aphrodisiac properties for centuries. Although it is possible that this is because they may have a direct hormonal influence, it is more likely that they work on a subtle level, influencing the mind and emotions through the sense of smell.

All essential oils are antiseptic. Some, such as eucalyptus, garlic and tea tree, have anti-viral properties as well. Unlike harsh chemical antiseptics, essential oils, if used correctly, act as powerful aggressors against germs without harming tissue.

When Dr Jean Valnet (see page 13) used essential oils to treat soldiers' wounds during the Second World War, not only did the fragrances mask the powerful odour of gangrenous wounds, the oils actively retarded putrefaction. Valnet also noticed that troops sleeping rough in pine forests suffered fewer respiratory complaints as a result of pine resin vapour saturating the air. For the same reason, Swiss sanatoriums are traditionally sited near pine forests to help patients suffering from chest conditions and tuberculosis.

What is the Chemistry of Essential Oils?
The chemistry of essential oils is complex. Unlike a synthetic drug which may contain a single, but very powerful active principle, an essential oil may consist of hundreds of components. For this reason, a single essence can help a wide variety of disorders (see Chapter 3).

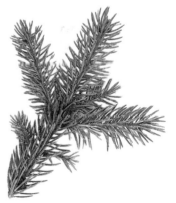

Valnet and other pioneers discovered that blends of certain essential oils act more powerfully than individual oils. This is especially noticeable with the anti-bacterial action of essences. For example, Valnet's blend of clove, thyme, lavender and peppermint produced a far more powerful effect than a chemist might expect from the combined chemical constituents of the oils. However, when one more oil was added to this blend, the effect was counter-productive because the anti-bacterial action becomes weaker.

Essential oils also act on the central nervous system. Some will relax (for example, camomile and rose), others will stimulate (for example, rosemary and black pepper). A few are able to 'normalize', or balance.

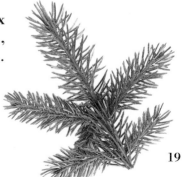

For example, when taken in capsule form, garlic can raise low blood pressure and lower high blood pressure. Similarly, bergamot and geranium can either sedate or stimulate according to individual needs. This pattern of 'balancing' healing is not achieved by synthetic drugs.

Studies have also shown that essential oils have a very small molecular structure, which enables them to pass through the skin's hair follicles. These follicles contain sebum, an oily liquid with which essential oils have an affinity. From here the essential oils diffuse into the bloodstream or are taken up by the lymph and interstitial fluid, a liquid surrounding all body cells, to other parts of the body. If the skin is healthy, it takes about thirty minutes for the oil to be absorbed; if the skin is congested or if there is much subcutaneous fat, it takes much longer. At the same time, when inhaled, the aromatic molecules reach the lungs from where they diffuse across tiny air sacs into the surrounding blood capillaries and then into the bloodstream.

Whether the oil is absorbed through the skin or inhaled, once in the bloodstream and body fluids, it works therapeutically – however small the dose. The actual efficacy of the oils may be due to the frequency of aromatherapy treatments which can be given once or twice weekly over a four-week period. Each session gently stimulates the body's self-healing ability and, once having triggered the healing process, the essential oils are rapidly eliminated, so if used correctly there is little danger of toxicity.

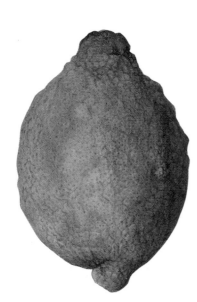

Sense of Smell

Researchers at Yale University, USA, have discovered that the aroma of apples and cinnamon has a powerful stabilizing effect on some people, especially those suffering from nervous anxiety. The smell has even been known to lower high blood pressure and to stave off panic attacks. How does this work?

The olfactory centre – the area of the brain associated with smell – merges with the limbic system which is concerned with basic drives such as hunger, thirst and sex and also with subtle responses such as emotion, memory, creativity and intuition. The olfactory area also connects to the hypothalamus, an important structure which influences the pituitary gland, and therefore controls the hormonal system.

From this it may be easier to understand how odours influence both the physical and emotional aspects of our being. Consider, for example, the aroma of your favourite food. The delicious vapour will stimulate your appetite by making your mouth water and at the same time cause the digestive juices to flow. If the aroma is associated with a happy occasion then memory comes into play as well, adding to the pleasurable rush.

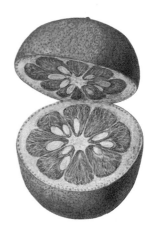

Pleasing aromas, along with enjoyments such as eating, falling in love, listening to music and looking at beautiful things, cause the release of certain 'happiness chemicals', which form part of a family of opium-like substances broadly labelled enkephalins and endorphins. Such release is found in chocolate and rosewater in the form of phenlethylamine. These 'happiness' substances are also known to help strengthen the immune system.

The power of aroma to conjure up memories is perhaps the most familiar. A mere hint of a certain scent may remind you of a first love, a special event or a childhood visit. Likewise certain aromas, no matter how pleasing to others, will evoke distressing feelings in somebody who associates the odour with an unpleasant experience. A friend of mine cannot abide the scent of jasmine because it reminds her of funerals. Another loathes the scent of rose because it reminds her of an unhappy episode at school, in particular a harsh schoolmistress who always smelled of a rose-scented perfume.

Many people also have 'blind spots' to certain odours, such as musks, or nuances of individual smells – an odour rarely arises from a single odoriferous molecule and is usually an interaction of many. Some people, however, can detect the merest hint of a particular odour.

Although a healthy olfactory centre can pick up over 10,000 different odours, if it is subjected to the same odour for even a short while, the olfactory cells become 'saturated', exhausted and cease to detect the odour, even though we may, from time to time, experience a fleeting reminder of its presence.

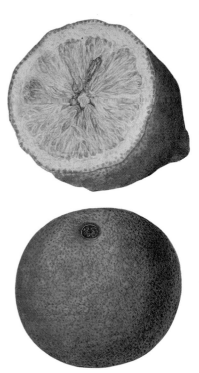

Of the many aroma trials carried out at Warwick University, England, by researchers Dr Steve Van Toller and Dr George Dodd, one was particularly notable. They produced evidence that we can respond both emotionally and physically to odours that are so highly diluted they are imperceptible to the conscious mind.

In the Van Toller-Dodd experiments, volunteers were wired up to an EEG (electro-encephalograph) instrument which records the brain's electrical activity along with subtle reactions of the skin. When they were exposed to low-level fragrance, very clear skin responses were noted. It appears that the skin acts like antennae, communicating the aroma to the body's central nervous system. Radiological scanning

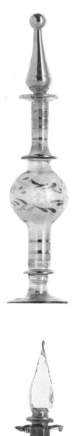

techniques also confirm the brain's registration of low-level fragrance.

From this we can consider that even sufferers of anosmia (major loss of the sense of smell) can benefit – albeit at a subtle level – from an aromatherapy treatment or perfume. Indeed, as mentioned earlier, whether we can continue to smell the oils or not during a treatment does not reduce the healing effect.

Personal Preferences

It was also discovered during the Van Toller-Dodd experiment that if we dislike an aroma we are able to block its effect on the central nervous system. This supports the case for using the oils we like best, especially for stress-related problems. Experience has also shown that we are instinctively drawn to the essential oil that is right for our needs at a given time. As our state of mind alters so may our preference.

Aroma choice is thought to be largely influenced by body odour which, in turn, is related to diet plus ethnic and genetic influences. Emotions, ill health, the Pill and other drugs, as well as hormonal changes caused by puberty, pregnancy and the menopause, also influence body odour and preferences.

This explains why the same perfume smells different on each person and why our choice varies when we select oils. As we age, our bodies secrete different *pheromones*, subliminal scent-chemicals, and, as a result, a favourite perfume in youth may seem far less attractive in maturity.

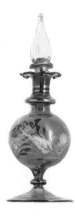

Aroma fashions also come and go. Valerian, for instance, was an extremely popular perfume in the sixteenth century – certainly it would have harmonized with odour of the infrequently washed bodies of the time. Indeed, valerian is considered more reminiscent of sweaty socks. Nowadays, its most loyal 'fans' are she-cats for whom it is said to be a potent aphrodisiac!

Aroma conditioning or fashion may also play a part in directing choice. Unfortunately this can be counter-productive when it inhibits personal needs and hinders the beneficial effects of essential oils. Essential oils are very different from synthetic perfumes and, for people not accustomed to them, may seem strange at first. However, once regularly used, the 'strangeness' wears off, revealing naturally beautiful aromas.

Natural Versus Synthetic

Although scientists have tried to duplicate essential oils in the laboratory, the results are not the same. A synthetic chemical is, in theory, identical to that found in nature, but in practice it is impossible to make a one hundred per cent pure chemical. Any synthetic chemical is bound to carry a small percentage of undesirable substances which are not found in the essential oil. Synthetic aromatic compounds also lack the vital enzymes and possibly a multitude of substances yet to be discovered in plants. In addition, aromatic chemicals smell differently from true essential oils and are more likely to cause allergies.

Buying Essential Oils

It is vital to use only pure, unadulterated essential oils in aromatherapy. Most aromatherapists obtain their oils from reputable mail order suppliers, not from shops concerned with beauty and perfumery. The advantages offered by mail order suppliers include a wider range of oils and lower prices on larger quantities. However, if you are new to aromatherapy, it may be best to buy your oils from a health shop or from a well-respected herbal supplier. This will give you the opportunity to smell the oils first, and buy only those that you like. But do check that an essential oil, labelled as such, is in fact one hundred per cent essential and has not been diluted in almond oil. This is sometimes the case with expensive oils such as rose otto or neroli.

Caring for Essential Oils

Storage is important. Essential oils should be sold in well-stoppered glass bottles and protected from heat and damp. Avoid essential oils in bottles with a rubber-tipped dropper (certain essential oils, cedarwood especially, can cause the rubber to dissolve). Despite this, essential oils are harmless to the skin when used in correct dilutions (see Chapter 4).

In theory, with the exception of citrus oils, most oils will keep for several years. However, although a citrus oil, bergamot essence will keep for up to two years. Some oils, such as sandalwood, frankincense, rose otto and patchouli mature with age rather like fine wines. A twenty-year-old patchouli essence will be extremely mellow and fragrant. However, the more frequently a bottle of essential oil is opened, the greater the chance of oxidation and thus a reduction in the oil's therapeutic properties. If stored in a cool dark place, essential oils will keep for at least one year. However, if diluted in vegetable oil for use in massage, essential oils will last for no more than two, possibly three months if stored correctly in a refrigerator.

Let's take a closer look at thirty of the most commonly used essential oils and their main therapeutic properties.

When selecting oils to help with anxiety and stress, choose fragrances that appeal to you. Aromatherapy is meant to be enjoyable – in fact, the more wonderful the experience, the greater the healing effect.

However, for the symptomatic treatment of conditions such as athlete's foot or sprains (see pages 114–117), aroma preference is probably less important. A bonus is that because each essential oil has a myriad of therapeutic properties, it is not too difficult to find an oil (or a blend of oils) to suit your aroma preference, as well as your physical and emotional needs. If, however, you are suffering from a deep-rooted problem, such as arthritis, asthma, eczema or chronic nervous tension, seek expert advice from a qualified practitioner, aromatherapist or counsellor, preferably someone with a knowledge of holistic healing principles. Diet and lifestyle play an important role in our physical and emotional well being.

Of course, you need not be injured, ill or stressed to enjoy aromatherapy – the oils can be used purely for pleasure. However, before using any essential oil, check that it is safe for you to do so. Some oils, especially those which stimulate menstruation, for example, should not be applied during pregnancy. Where appropriate, a caution note is included at the end of each essential oil profile.

Allergies

It is possible to be allergic to almost anything – even to the seemingly innocuous sweet almond oil. A few people may be skin-sensitive to oils such as basil, bergamot, geranium, ginger, lemongrass, melissa, peppermint and ylang-ylang, especially in high concentrations. If you are one of the rare people allergic to all essential oils, you will have to try another therapy such as homoeopathy or herbal medicine. However, you can still enjoy giving and receiving massage by using plain vegetable oil rather than an aromatherapy blend.

CAUTION
* *Essential oils are very powerful, so need to be used with care.*
* *During pregnancy, whilst breastfeeding, and for children under twelve years old, it is advisable to use oils in half the stated quantities.*
* *Never use essential oils for babies or young children except under the strict guidance of a qualified aromatherapist.*
* *Never use an essential oil about which you can find little or no information.*
* *Never take essential oils internally.*
* *If you suffer from asthma, never use steam inhalations, with or without essential oils. Concentrated steam may trigger an attack.*
Recommended concentrations for essential oils are given on pages 38–39

Basil

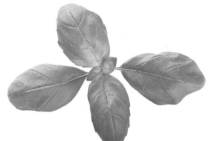

(Ocymum basilicum)

SOURCE
Distillation of the leaves and flowering tops from this herb which is native to the Far East and Africa.

AROMA
Agreeably spicy, vaguely reminiscent of cloves.

BLENDS WELL WITH
Bergamot and other citrus oils, frankincense, geranium, neroli.

USES
Primarily a nerve tonic and a mental stimulant. Helps bronchitis, colds, coughs, headache, mental and physical fatigue, menstruation (scanty), sinus problems.

Caution
Do not use during pregnancy. Avoid if you have sensitive skin. Always use in the lowest concentrations.

Bergamot

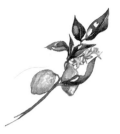

(Citrus bergamia)

SOURCE
Obtained by expressing the rind of the small orange-like fruit native to Italy.

AROMA
Delightfully citrus with a slightly spicy overtone.

BLENDS WELL WITH
Most other essences, particularly coriander, geranium, lavender, vetiver, ylang-ylang.

USES
Primarily uplifting and anti-depressant. A 'balancing' oil capable of relaxing or stimulating, according to individual needs. Helpful for boils, cold sores, cystitis, fevers, oily skin conditions, pre-menstrual syndrome, and tonsillitis (as a gargle: put four drops in a teacup of warm water and use two or three times a day).

Caution
Do not use on the skin immediately before sunbathing, as it may cause temporary pigmentation. However it is now possible to obtain bergaptene-free bergamot essence, labelled 'Bergamot FCF', which will not react with the skin in sunlight. As a skin oil, it is advisable to use this essence in a moderate to low concentration.

Black Pepper

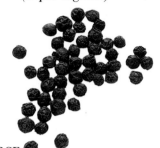

(Piper nigrum)

SOURCE
Steam distillation of the dried-and-crushed black peppercorns from the fruit of the woody vine, native of India.

AROMA
Warm, dry-woody and peppery.

BLENDS WELL WITH
Coriander, frankincense, ginger, lavender, marjoram, rosemary, rose otto, sandalwood, ylang-ylang.

USES
Reputed to be an aphrodisiac, and stimulant. Helpful for appetite (loss of), chilblains, circulation (poor), colic, constipation, coughs and colds, diarrhoea, infections and viruses, influenza, lethargy, muscular aches and pains, nausea, neuralgia.

Caution
Best avoided during the first three months of pregnancy as the oil may be too stimulating.

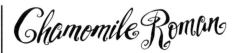

Cedarwood
(Juniperus viginiana)

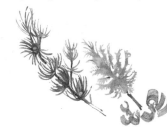

SOURCE
Distillation of the wood shavings from the evergreen tree native to North America.

AROMA
Woody, reminiscent of pencils!

BLENDS WELL WITH
Bergamot, clary sage, cypress, juniper, neroli, rose, rosemary, vetiver, ylang-ylang.

USES
Acts primarily on the skin and the respiratory tract; has diuretic properties. Reputed to be an aphrodisiac. Helpful for acne, anxiety, bronchitis, catarrh, coughs, cystitis, dandruff, eczema (use in half per cent concentrations), oily skin conditions, pre-menstrual syndrome, and as an insect repellent.

Caution
Do not use during pregnancy.

Chamomile Roman
(Chamaemelum nobile syn. Anthemis noblis)

SOURCE
Distillation of the dried daisy-like flowers from the herb native to northern Europe. It is not to be confused with the cheaper Moroccan chamomile (Ormenis multicaulis). Although distantly related to Roman chamomile and, with a similar aroma, Moroccan chamomile's value as a healing agent is regarded as inferior.

AROMA
Dry and slightly sweet with an herbaceous undertone.

BLENDS WELL WITH
Citrus essences, geranium, lavender, rose, ylang-ylang.

USES
Primarily an anti-inflammatory (due to a high content of chamazulene), and a sedative. Helpful for acne, allergies (skin and respiratory), anxiety, boils, chilblains, cold sores, colic, colitis, ear infections, eczema, indigestion, inflammation of joints, insomnia, menopausal problems, menstruation (painful), migraine, neuralgia, pre-menstrual syndrome, psoriasis, rheumatism, skin care (most skins), sprains, stomach cramps, swellings, thread veins, wounds.

Caution
A very powerful essence which is best used in the lowest concentrations, especially when treating allergies.

Clary Sage
(Salvia sclarea)

SOURCE
Distillation of the flowering leaves and tops from the herb native to the Mediterranean.

AROMA
Sweet and warmly floral, very different from the herby aroma of common sage (Salvia officinalis).

BLENDS WELL WITH
Cedarwood, citrus essences, cypress, frankincense, geranium, lavender, marjoram, neroli, peppermint, petitgrain, sandalwood.

USES
Primarily as a warming and relaxing nerve tonic. Reputed to be an aphrodisiac. Helpful for absence of periods outside pregnancy, anxiety, boils, excessive perspiration, high blood pressure, insect bites and stings, insomnia, leucorrhoea (vaginal discharge), menstruation (painful), nervous tension, pre-menstrual syndrome, throat infections, whooping cough.

Caution
Do not use during pregnancy.

Coriander

(Coriandrum sativum)

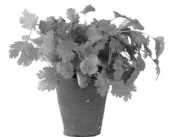

SOURCE
Distillation of the fruit (the so-called seeds) of a herb indigenous to southern Europe.

AROMA
Agreeably piquant and fruity.

BLENDS WELL WITH
Citrus oils, cypress, juniper, marjoram, petitgrain.

USES
Generally warming and stimulating to the mind, it was formerly held to be an aphrodisiac. Helpful for colic, depression, loss of appetite, mental fatigue, nervous debility, rheumatism.

Cypress

(Cupressus sempervirens)

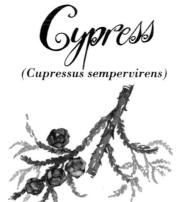

SOURCE
Distillation of the leaves and fruit (cones) of the tall, conical-shaped tree native to the East and the Mediterranean.

AROMA
Cooling, somewhat solemn, similar to pine.

BLENDS WELL WITH
Cedarwood, citrus oils, clary sage, lavender, marjoram, myrrh, petitgrain, pine needle, sandalwood.

USES
Primarily astringent, mentally clearing and mildly sedative. Helpful for anxiety and nervous tension, bronchitis, cellulite, diarrhoea, excessive perspiration, haemorrhoids, incontinence, influenza, loss of voice, menopausal problems, menstruation (heavy and painful), oily skin conditions, pyorrhoea, rheumatism, spasmodic coughs, thread veins, varicose veins.

Eucalyptus

(Eucalyptus globulus)

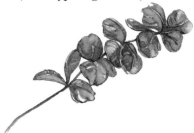

SOURCE
Distillation of the leaves of a tall tree native to Australia.

AROMA
Camphoric.

BLENDS WELL WITH
Lavender, lemon, peppermint, pine, sandalwood.

USES
A powerful antiseptic with a marked effect on the respiratory system. Helpful for allergies to animal fur; bronchitis, burns, catarrh, cold sores, colds, coughs, cystitis, diabetes (can lower excess blood sugar levels), fevers, hayfever, head lice, influenza, leucorrhoea (vaginal discharge), measles, migraine, neuralgia, rheumatism, scarlet fever, sinusitis, sprains, throat infections, ulcers of the skin, wounds, and as an insect repellent.

Frankincense

(Boswellia thurifera)

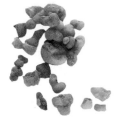

SOURCE
Distillation of the hardened resin ('tears') of the small north African countries tree.

AROMA
Warm and balsamic.

BLENDS WELL WITH
Basil, black pepper, cedarwood, citrus essences, coriander, lavender, myrrh, neroli, rose, sandalwood, vetiver.

USES
Highly valued for its effects on the mind, especially when used as an aid to meditation, and for its effect on the respiratory tract. Helpful for acne, bronchitis, catarrh, coughs, deep wounds, haemorrhoids, lethargy, nose bleeds, skin care (particularly ageing skin).

Geranium

(Peiargonium odoratissimum)

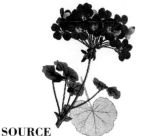

SOURCE
Distillation of the whole plant native to Reunion, Madagascar and Guinea.

AROMA
Freshly floral and sweet.

BLENDS WELL WITH
Most other essences, especially bergamot, neroli, petitgrain, ylang-ylang.

USES
Like bergamot, geranium is a balancing essence, capable of relaxing or stimulating according to individual needs. Helpful for cellulite, diabetes (like eucalyptus, it can lower excessive blood sugar levels), fluid retention, mouth ulcers, neuralgia, ringworm, shingles, sore throats, thrush, wounds.

Caution
Although a balancing oil for most people, this oil may be too stimulating for a few sensitive individuals. Moreover, mothers who have used the oil on their skin when breastfeeding have reported that it sometimes has a stimulating effect on babies.

Ginger

(Zingiber officinale)

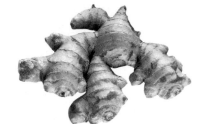

SOURCE
Distillation of the roots (rhizomes) of the plant native to China.

AROMA
Not as pleasantly pungent as the freshly-grated root. Unfortunately, the intense heat of distillation tends to distort the aroma.

BLENDS WELL WITH
Citrus oils, coriander, patchouli, vetiver. But use sparingly, otherwise its powerful aroma will dominate the blends.

USES
Warming for both body and mind. A reputed aphrodisiac. Helpful for anxiety and nervous tension, arthritis, chilblains, colds, cramp, fibrositis, influenza, muscle sprain, muscular aches and pains, poor circulation, rheumatism, and as a gargle for sore throats (one or two drops in a cup of water, stir well).

Caution
Unsuitable for those with sensitive skin. Avoid during pregnancy as it may be too stimulating.

Grapefruit
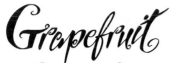

(Citrus x paradisi)

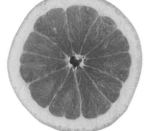

SOURCE
Expressed from the skin of the fruit of the tree native to tropical Asia, but cultivated elsewhere, especially California. An inferior grade oil, with a somewhat murky aroma, is distilled from the peel and remains of the fruit after the juice has been utilized, so always ask for the expressed oil.

AROMA
Fresh, sweet and citrus.

BLENDS WELL WITH
Other citrus essences, coriander (and other spices), cypress, geranium, lavender, neroli, rosemary.

USES
Primarily uplifting and anti-depressant, it is helpful for anxiety and depression, cellulite, colds and influenza, fluid retention, nervous exhaustion, performance stress.

Caution
*Do not use on the skin immediately before sunbathing, as it may cause temporary pigmentation.
It has a short shelf life, so buy small quantities and use within six months.*

Juniper

(Juniperus communis)

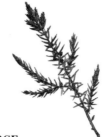

SOURCE
Distillation of the berries from the evergreen shrub native to the northern hemisphere.

AROMA
Astringent, slightly peppery, with a resinous overtone.

BLENDS WELL WITH
Citrus essences, geranium, lavender, myrrh, rosemary, sandalwood.

USES
Primarily cleansing and diuretic, it is also used as a tonic. Helpful for absence of periods outside pregnancy, arthritis, cellulite, coughs, cystitis, fluid retention, gout, haemorrhoids, loss of appetite, nervous tension, oily skin conditions, respiratory infections, rheumatism, weeping eczema.

Caution
Do not use during pregnancy. Try to obtain the top-grade oil labelled 'Juniper Berry' rather than 'Juniper' – the latter is usually an inferior oil distilled from the twigs rather than the fruit.

Lavender

(Lavandula angustifolia)

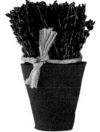

SOURCE
Distillation of the leaves and flowering tops of the plant native to the Mediterranean.

AROMA
Refreshingly floral with a balsamic, woody undertone.

BLENDS WELL WITH
Most other essences, especially bergamot, chamomile, clary sage, frankincense, grapefruit, juniper, marjoram, rose, vetiver, ylang-ylang.

USES
Regulates the central nervous system. Helpful for abscesses, acne, anxiety, athlete's foot, boils, bronchitis, burns, chilblains, colds, coughs, cuts, cystitis, dandruff, depression, earache, eczema, fainting, flatulence, fluctuating moods, head lice, high blood pressure, infectious illness, insect bites and stings, insomnia, laryngitis, leucorrhoea (vaginal discharge), menstruation (scanty and painful), migraine, muscular aches and pains, nervous tension, pre-menstrual syndrome, skin care (all skin types), sprains, and as a hair tonic.

Lemon
(Citrus limonum)

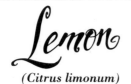

SOURCE
Expressing of the lemon rind of the lemon tree native to the Mediterranean.

AROMA
Clear, sharp, refreshing. The essential oil does not keep well; use within six-to-nine months.

BLENDS WELL WITH
Most other essences, especially chamomile, eucalyptus, frankincense, geranium, juniper, lavender, pine, ylang-ylang.

USES
Fortifying to the nervous system, and helpful for anaemia, arthritis, cellulite, chilblains, colds, fluid retention, gallstones, high blood pressure, influenza, insect bites and stings, rheumatism, sore throats, verrucae, warts, wounds, and as an insect repellent.

Caution
Do not use on the skin prior to sunbathing. It may cause temporary pigmentation. Can also cause skin irritation if used in high concentrations.

Marjoram, Sweet
(Origanum majorana)

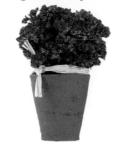

SOURCE
Distillation of the flowering tops and leaves from the herb native to Hungary.

AROMA
Warm, camphoric and vaguely spicy.

BLENDS WELL WITH
Bergamot, chamomile, coriander, cypress, cedarwood, eucalyptus, lavender, peppermint, rosemary.

USES
Has a warming and calming effect on the nervous system. Helpful for anxiety and nervous tension, arthritis, bronchitis, bruises, colds, constipation, flatulence, headaches, high blood pressure, indigestion, leucorrhoea (vaginal discharge), menstruation (painful), migraine, muscular aches and pains.

Caution
Do not use during pregnancy.

Myrrh
(Commiphora myrrha)

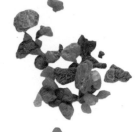

SOURCE
Steam distillation of the hardened myrrh exudes or 'tears' from the shrub or small tree native to southwest Asia and the Red Sea region.

AROMA
Rather medicinal, warm and balsamic.

BLENDS WELL WITH
Cypress, frankincense, geranium, juniper, lavender, lemon, patchouli, pine, sandalwood.

USES
An anti-catarrhal, anti-inflammatory with pronounced anti-fungal properties. Its action on the nervous system is sedative, yet it also stimulates digestion and menstruation and is a good expectorant. Helpful for arthritis, athlete's foot, coughs and colds, cracked skin, gum infections, menstruation (loss of outside pregnancy), mouth ulcers, respiratory disorders, ringworm, sore throat, voice (loss of), wounds.

Caution
Do not use during pregnancy. Myrrh oil tends to thicken slightly on contact with the air, so, before use, steep the bottle in a cup of warm water for a few minutes until the oil reaches dropping consistency.

Neroli or Orange Blossom

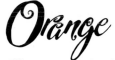

(Citrus aurantium)

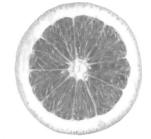

SOURCE
Distillation of the blossom from the bitter orange tree native to China and extensively cultivated in southern Europe, California and Florida.

AROMA
Bitter-sweet, not at all 'citrusy'.

BLENDS WELL WITH
Most essences, especially bergamot (and other citrus oils) chamomile, clary sage, coriander, geranium, lavender, rose, ylang-ylang.

USES
Primarily as an anti-depressant and sedative with a slightly hypnotic effect, at least for some individuals. Reputed to be an aphrodisiac. Helpful for depression, emotional shock, hyperanxiety, insomnia, nervous tension, palpitations, pre-menstrual syndrome, skin care (suitable for most skin types, has a toning effect).

Orange

(Citrus aurantium)

(Oil of Mandarin, Citrus nobilis and also Tangerine, Citrus reticulata, have similar, although less pronounced properties, and a sweeter, more delicate aroma.)

SOURCE
Expressing of the rind from the fruit native to China; also extensively cultivated in southern Europe, California and Florida.

AROMA
Similar to fresh oranges (or it should be if the oil is fresh!), sweet and uplifting. The essential oil of most citrus fruits (except bergamot) does not keep well, so use within six-to-nine months of purchase.

BLENDS WELL WITH
Most oils, including other citrus essences, clary sage, coriander (and all other spices), cypress, frankincense, geranium, juniper, lavender, rose, vetiver, ylang-ylang.

USES
As a general tonic with an uplifting aroma. Helpful for anxiety and depression, bronchitis, chills, colds, palpitations.

Caution
Do not apply to the skin prior to sunbathing. It may cause temporary pigmentation.

Patchouli

(Pogostemon patchouli)

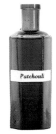

SOURCE
Distillation of the dried leaves from the herb native to the tropical Far East.

AROMA
An earthy Eastern scent which becomes sweeter once the sour element of the oil has worn off – improves with age.

BLENDS WELL WITH
Cedarwood, citrus essences, clary sage, geranium, ginger, lavender, neroli, rose, sandalwood.

USES
Primarily antibiotic, anti-fungal, anti-depressant and fortifying. Reputed to be an aphrodisiac. Helpful for acne, anxiety and depression, athlete's foot, cellulite, cracked skin, dandruff, depression, fevers, fluid retention, hair-thinning, sores, wounds.

Peppermint

(Mentha x piperita)

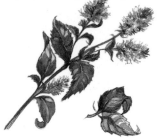

SOURCE
Steam distillation of the flowering tops of the herb native to Europe and parts of Asia.

AROMA
Piercing, grassy-minty.

BLENDS WELL WITH
Because it has such a powerful aroma, it does not blend well with other essences, although it is acceptable in tiny quantities with clary sage, eucalyptus, lavender, lemon, marjoram, rosemary.

USES
A cooling, mentally stimulating oil. Helpful for catarrh, colds, flatulence, indigestion, influenza, migraine, muscular aches and pains, nausea, neuralgia, ringworm, scabies, sinusitis, toothache (as a first-aid measure, apply a few drops to the tooth cavity and around the gum).

Caution
Use the lowest concentration as it may irritate sensitive skin. Avoid during the first three months of pregnancy as it may be too stimulating.

Petitgrain

(Citrus aurantium)

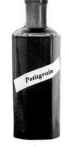

SOURCE
Distillation of the leaves and twigs of the bitter orange tree native to China; also extensively cultivated in southern Europe, California and Florida.

AROMA
Similar to neroli, but less refined with a woody-herbaceous undertone.

BLENDS WELL WITH
Bergamot and other citrus essences, clary sage, cypress, geranium, juniper, lavender, pine, rosemary, ylang-ylang.

USES
Primarily for fortifying the nervous system. Helpful for anxiety and nervous tension, convalescence, insomnia, palpitations.

Pine Scots

(Pinus sylvestris)

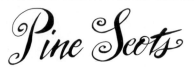

SOURCE
Distillation of the pine needles of the tree native to northern Europe. The highest grade oil is obtained from the needles. Lower grades are obtained by distillation of the cones, young twigs and branches.

AROMA
Cooling and woody with a dry balsamic overtone.

BLENDS WELL WITH
Bergamot and other citrus essences, cedarwood, cypress, geranium, juniper, lavender, patchouli, petitgrain, rosemary, sandalwood.

USES
Primarily antiseptic, antibiotic, diuretic and stimulating, and also an expectorant. Helpful for arthritis, bronchitis, catarrh, colds, cystitis, influenza, laryngitis, lethargy, rheumatism, wounds.

Caution
Use in low dilutions as it can cause irritation to sensitive skin.

Rose Otto
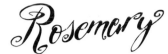
(Rosa damascena)

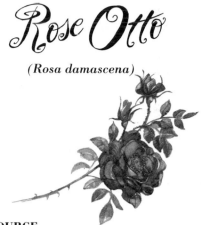

SOURCE
Distillation of the flower petals of the plant native to Bulgaria.

AROMA
Smooth and warm with a hint of vanilla and cloves. Not to be confused with rose absolute (extracted by solvents), which is yellowy-orange and has a lighter aroma. Rose Otto is virtually colourless and is semi-solid at room temperature.

BLENDS WELL WITH
Many essences, especially bergamot and other citrus oils, cedarwood, chamomile, clary sage, frankincense, lavender, patchouli, sandalwood, ylang-ylang. A tiny amount is all you will need as it is highly odoriferous.

USES
Primarily an oil for healing distressing states of mind such as anxiety and depression. The essence is reputed to be an aphrodisiac. Also helpful for gynaecological disorders, hangover (it has a cleansing effect on the liver), leucorrhoea (vaginal discharge), menopausal symptoms, menstruation (heavy and irregular), pre-menstrual syndrome, respiratory disorders, skin care (especially dry, ageing skin), thread veins.

Rosemary
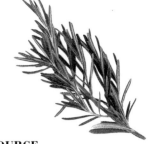
(Rosmarinus officinalis)

SOURCE
Distillation of the flowering tops of the herb native to the Mediterranean.

AROMA
Warm, sharp and camphoric.

BLENDS WELL WITH
Basil, cedarwood, citrus oils, coriander (and other spices), frankincense, juniper, lavender, petitgrain, pine.

USES
Primarily a stimulating essence for both body and mind. Helpful for arthritis, bronchitis, burns, cholesterol (high), colds, dandruff, hair-thinning, head lice, headache, indigestion, influenza, low blood pressure, mental fatigue, migraine, nervous debility, palpitations, rheumatism, skin care (especially oily skin), wounds.

Caution
Do not use during the first three months of pregnancy as it may be too stimulating. In very high concentrations, and if used continuously over a long period of time, it may provoke convulsions in people who are prone to these.

Sandalwood
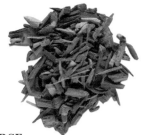
(Santalum album)

SOURCE
Distillation of the heart, or soft wood found under the bark of the tree. Native to India, sandalwood is a small parasitic tree (it buries its roots in those of neighbouring trees). The so-called West Indian sandalwood or amyris balsamifera is a poor substitute and bears no botanical relation to the East Indian sandalwood.

AROMA
Deep, softly woody and sweet, of excellent tenacity.

BLENDS WELL WITH
Many essences, especially bergamot, frankincense, geranium, patchouli, rose, ylang-ylang.

USES
Primarily for urinary tract infections, nervous tension, respiratory disorders and skin problems. Reputed to be an aphrodisiac. Helpful for acne, bronchitis, catarrh, coughs, cystitis, depression, diarrhoea, insomnia, laryngitis, pre-menstrual syndrome, skin care (oily, dry or ageing skins).

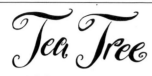

Tea Tree
(Melaleuca alternifolia)

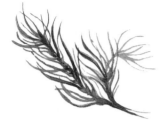

SOURCE
Distillation of the leaves and twigs of the hardy tree native to Australia.

AROMA
Medicinal, reminiscent of a mixture of juniper and cypress, but less refined than these two oils.

BLENDS WELL WITH
It does not blend well with other essences, but the aroma can be improved by mixing with a little eucalyptus, lemon, lavender or pine.

USES
Primarily an antiseptic, antibiotic, anti-viral, anti-fungal essence. A powerful immune system stimulant. Helpful for acne, athlete's foot, cold sores, colds, coughs, dandruff, influenza, insect bites and stings, ringworm, thrush, verrucae, warts, wounds. A few drops in the bath can soothe the effects of hyperanxiety.

Caution
Can cause temporary irritation to sensitive skin.

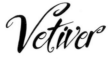

Vetiver
(Vetiveria zizanioides)

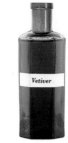

SOURCE
Steam distillation of the roots of a tall, scented grass native to India.

AROMA
Rich, earthy and sweet, reminiscent of molasses.

BLENDS WELL WITH
clary sage, lavender, patchouli, rose, sandalwood, ylang-ylang.

USES
Primarily an oil for healing distressing states of mind such as anxiety, insomnia, nervous tension and stress. Also helpful for acne, arthritis, circulation (poor), rheumatism, muscular aches and pains, oily skin conditions, wounds.

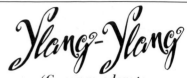

Ylang-Ylang
(Cananga odorata, pronounced ee-lang-ee-lang)

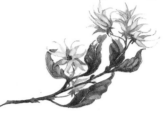

SOURCE
Distillation of the flower petals of the tree native to tropical Asia. There are several grades of ylang-ylang, so always obtain the higher priced oil labelled 'ylang-ylang extra'. Other grades are less refined and lack the special creamy richness of the top-quality essence.

AROMA
Intensely sweet, soft, floral-balsamic, reminiscent of the scent of almonds and jasmine combined.

BLENDS WELL WITH
Cedarwood, chamomile, citrus oils, geranium, lavender, patchouli, rose, sandalwood.

USES
Primarily an oil for healing distressing emotions, and to slow down over-rapid breathing and heartbeat. Reputed to be an aphrodisiac. Helpful for anxiety, depression, high blood pressure, nervous tension, palpitations, pre-menstrual syndrome, shock.

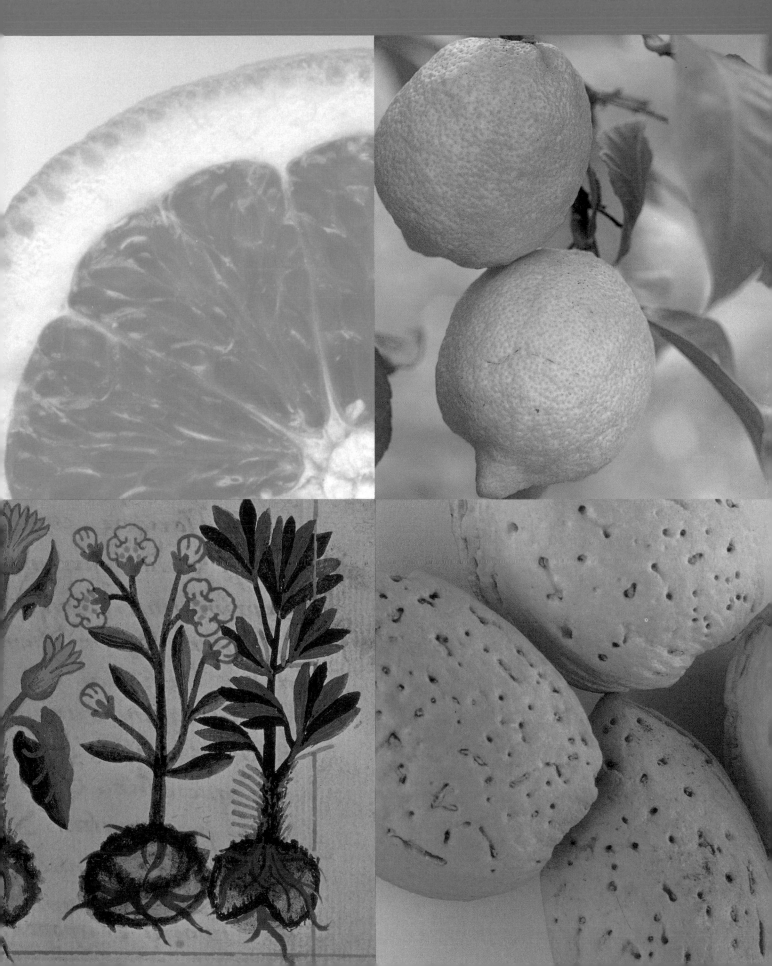

There are many enjoyable ways to use essential oils to alleviate health problems and to create a sense of well-being. Pride of place must go to aromatherapy massage, one of the finest treatments available to soothe all kinds of distress (see Chapter 5). But first let's look at the basics of aromatherapy, such as the blending of massage oils, fragrant creams and perfumes, and how these are applied.

Selecting Essential Oils

The oils profiled in Chapter 3 tend to be the most popular with aromatherapists. However, it would be extremely costly to buy them all at once. For the beginner, about six carefully-chosen oils will certainly be enough.

Although aroma preference affects our assessment of a blend of oils, do not be put off by an essence that is not immediately attractive. You may discover that it smells wonderful when used in tiny quantities and blended with other essences. Patchouli and vetiver are good examples. On first acquaintance their heavy, earthy, definitely Eastern aromas may seem overpowering, but blend them with larger quantities of more familiar fragrances such as bergamot, lavender and geranium and a synthesis takes place, creating a successful marriage of opposites.

Ideally any initial selection of essences will include a representative from each of the aroma families listed opposite. Those in italics were not mentioned in the previous chapter, but are certainly worth considering.

Base Oils

Essential oils, intended for massage, need to be diluted in a fine-quality, preferably unrefined or cold-pressed vegetable oil, such as almond, apricot kernel or sunflower seed. If an oil is not labelled as unrefined or cold-pressed, it is certain to be a refined product extracted by a process of high-pressure, intense heat and possibly even chemical solvents.

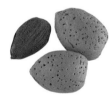

Unlike refined oils, such as those labelled simply 'vegetable oil', unrefined oils are rich in fat-soluble nutrients and essential fatty acids which can be easily absorbed through the skin and utilized by the body. Even without the addition of essential oils, these vegetable oils are health treatments in themselves. Extra virgin olive oil, for example, can sometimes help calm inflamed skin, and can be used as a massage oil for arthritic complaints.

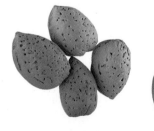

Aroma Families Chart

Ideally, any initial selection of essences will include a representative from each of the aroma families listed below. Those in italics were not mentioned in Chapter 3, but are certainly worth considering.

BALSAMIC OR RESINOUS	Frankincense, *galbanum*, myrrh **Caution:** *myrrh should not be used during pregnancy.*
CITRUS	Bergamot, grapefruit, lemon, *lime*, *mandarin*, orange
EARTHY	Patchouli, vetiver
FLORAL	Geranium, lavender, neroli (orange blossom), rose, ylang-ylang **Hint:** *If you like the aroma of neroli, but find the price prohibitive, try the much cheaper, but similar-smelling petitgrain, which is distilled from the leaves of the orange tree. The aroma is much less refined than that of its floral sister, but acceptable as a background note in blends.*
HERBAL	Basil, chamomile, clary sage, marjoram, rosemary
MEDICINAL	Eucalyptus, tea tree
PINE-LIKE	Cypress, juniper, pine
SPICY	Black pepper, *cardamom*, *cinnamon bark*, *clove*, coriander, ginger **Caution:** *Cinnamon and clove oils should never be used on the skin, as they can be highly irritant. Use only to perfume rooms.*
WOODY	Cedarwood, sandalwood

The woody, pine-like and medicinal families can be grouped together, partly because they are from trees and also because they tend to blend well with each other, albeit in a rather conservative way.

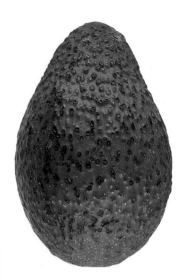

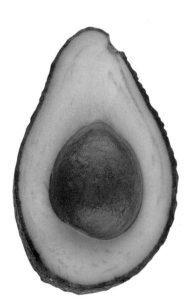

Mineral oil (baby oil) derives from petroleum and is to be avoided if you do not wish to use synthetic products. It lacks the beneficial properties of unrefined vegetable oils, and, when rubbed on the skin or swallowed, can cause vitamins A and E to leach from the body. It also tends to clog the pores contributing to the formation of blackheads and spots. Last but not least, the use of any type of synthetic oil runs counter to the philosophy of aromatherapy.

Most aromatherapists favour bland base oils, such as almond or grapeseed, the latter being only obtainable as a refined oil, because such oils do not impart their own aroma to the fragrant blends. However, the faintly nutty odour of unrefined vegetable oil, or the pungency of virgin olive oil, can blend harmoniously with the aromas of essential oils. For a cheaper, less pungent or nutty concoction, mix a refined oil such as grapeseed with an equal, or smaller, amount of an unrefined oil like extra virgin olive, sunflower seed or sesame. Please note that the dark sesame oil comes from toasted seeds and is too strong for use in aromatherapy – unless you relish smelling like a stir-fry!

For a facial oil, apricot kernel is one of the lightest to use, while avocado is very rich and highly penetrative – superb for dry or mature skins. Jojoba (pronounced ho-ho-ba), a liquid wax, is another popular oil. It is extracted from a small, evergreen plant native to the deserts of South America. Jojoba can even be used on oily or acneous skin, as a carrier for essential oils. In this instance, any excess oil can be tissued off after about thirty minutes once the essences have taken effect. To cut costs, these more expensive base oils can be diluted with a quantity of a cheaper oil such as almond or grapeseed.

Grapeseed oil and unrefined or cold-pressed vegetable oils are available from health shops and some supermarkets. Speciality oils, like avocado and jojoba, are easier to buy through mail order from most essential oil suppliers (see addresses in the Appendix).

Mixing Massage Oils

First choose the essential oil, or oils, to suit your physical and/or emotional needs. To do this, refer to the therapeutic charts in Chapter 7 and the essential oil profiles in Chapter 3. If you wish to prepare a facial oil suitable for your skin type, see page 39.

Essential oils need to be diluted at a rate of half-to-three per cent (see Easy Measures opposite). The ratios depend on a person's skin, the strength of the essential oil and the condition for which it is required.

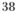

The lowest concentrations, half-to-one per cent, are best for the facial oils, young children and those with sensitive skin. If you have sensitive skin, it is best to start with half per cent concentration and, if this causes no irritation, increase to one per cent. For a body oil gradually build up to two per cent. Even for those with so-called normal skin, concentrations above two-and-a-half per cent are rarely advisable for massage, except in cases of great muscular tension when three per cent ratios of certain oils can be effective.

CAUTION

A few oils are very strong, or highly odoriferous, and should always be used in concentrations no greater than half-to-one per cent. These include basil, chamomile, fennel, ginger, lemongrass, melissa and peppermint. Black pepper, citrus oils, geranium, neroli and ylang-ylang are also best used in concentrations no higher than one-and-a-half to two per cent for body massage, for, in higher concentrations, these too can irritate very sensitive skins.

Although very expensive, rose otto has a strong aroma which means a tiny amount will go a long way. Again you will rarely need more than half-to-one per cent concentration of this essence.

Easy Measures

To mix enough oil for one massage, use a 5ml plastic medicine spoon to measure the base oil. An ordinary teaspoon will do, but can be smaller.

Preparing a Facial Oil

For a half per cent concentration, add one drop of essential oil to every two teaspoons of base oil. For a one per cent mix, add one drop of essential oil to each teaspoon of base oil. For a two per cent concentration, add two drops of essential oil to each teaspoon of base oil. However, do not exceed a two per cent concentration when preparing facial oils.

Preparing a Body Oil

For each two or three per cent concentration, add two or three drops of essential oil to each teaspoon of base oil. For larger quantities of massage oil, fill a 50ml dark-glass bottle with a base oil, then add the required amount of essential oil. For a half per cent concentration, add five drops to every 50ml of base oil. For a one per cent concentration in the same amount of base oil, add ten drops of essential oil; for a two per cent concentration, add thirty drops. Store in a cool, dark place, but use within a couple of months.

Skin Care

A healthy skin is a reflection of general well-being. No amount of external treatment with the finest plant oils, will help much if your diet, lifestyle and emotions are out of balance. Bear this in mind when treating your skin, and the oils will work more efficiently, adding far more than just the sheen.

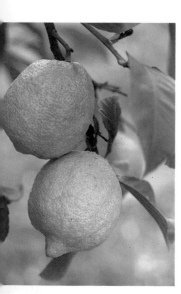

Even if you are one of the lucky few, blessed with a trouble-free skin, the use of essential oils and other non-synthetic preparations will help to preserve your skin's suppleness for as long as possible. Since the aromatic molecules of plant essences penetrate the skin's deepest layers, and end up in the bloodstream, they can have a positively profound effect. They nourish, tone, detoxify, soothe and generally support the skin's functions.

Essential oils used in baths (see page 41) and general massage also help the complexion, even when they are not applied directly to the face. For example, although very congested or oily skin cannot absorb essences efficiently, when essences are used in baths and general massage they are easily absorbed through the softer skin of the abdomen, inner thighs and upper arms, and by inhalation of the fragrant vapours. In this way, essential oils work systemically to influence the body as a whole.

Using Aromatherapy Facial Oils

The most beneficial way to use an aromatherapy facial oil is to apply it as a periodic treatment; either once a week, or daily for two weeks with a three-to-four week interval. This prevents the skin from becoming too used to the essences and thus failing to respond positively to them.

Choose an appropriate essential oil for your skin condition by referring to the skin care chart on page 42, then prepare a facial oil as described previously. There are various ways of applying the oils for maximum results.

1. *Apply a thin film just after bathing or showering when the skin is still warm and moist. Leave on for twenty minutes to allow for full absorption before wiping off any excess.*
2. *Apply thirty minutes after a facepack or facial sauna. The skin needs to settle down after such treatments so it can absorb the oils more efficiently.*
3. *Apply shortly before a walk in the fresh air. The combination of oxygen and essential oils is a superb skin rejuvenator.*

If you opt for a once-a-week regime, apply the oils three times a day, otherwise one daily application is enough.

Instead of using a facial oil, you may prefer to adapt an unperfumed face cream or lotion, preferably a plant-based product free of mineral oil. These are obtainable from some essential oil suppliers. Use the appropriate essence for your skin type. Stir in two-to-three drops of essential oil to 30g of face cream or one-to-two drops to 25ml of lotion and shake well.

Facial Sauna

This method can be used as a facial-cleansing treatment. Most skin types benefit from a weekly or fortnightly steaming with essential oils. It is particularly good for blemished and clogged skin, but should be avoided by people prone to thread veins. The intense heat dilates the blood vessels lying under the skin's surface and exacerbates the condition.

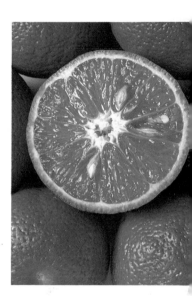

Put one or two drops of a suitable essence (see page 42) into a bowl containing half a litre of steaming water. Cover your whole head with a towel and put it over the steaming bowl, so the towel forms a tent to hold the steam. Stay inside for up to five minutes. Finish the treatment by splashing your face with cool water to remove the waste deposits accumulated on your skin's surface. Wait fifteen-to-twenty minutes before applying a moisturiser or aromatherapy facial oil.

Aromatic Baths

Essences can be added to your bath simply for pleasure, to aid restful sleep, to help skin disorders, relieve muscular and other pains, or to subtly influence your mood. They can be used singly, or blended with other essences.

Sprinkle three-to-six drops of essential oil on to the water's surface after the bath has been drawn. Agitate the water to disperse the oil. If you add essential oils as the water is running, much of the aromatic vapour will have evaporated before you get into the bath. If you have dry skin, mix the essences with a few teaspoons of vegetable oil. For a more soluble mixture, mix the oils with a dessertspoon of mild, unperfumed liquid soap or shampoo. Children can benefit from aromatic baths, too, but do not use more than three drops of essential oil to an average-size bath. Never use essences for babies unless under the strict guidance of a qualified aromatherapist.

Skincare Chart

SKIN TYPE	RECOMMENDED OILS
Dry Skin	Chamomile, lavender, neroli, rose otto, sandalwood, ylang-ylang
Oily Skin	Bergamot, cedarwood, cypress, eucalyptus, frankincense, geranium, juniper, lavender, lemon, patchouli, rosemary, tea tree
'Normal' Skin	Chamomile, frankincense, geranium, lavender, neroli, rose otto
Ageing Skin	Frankincense, rose otto, sandalwood
Puffy Skin	Cypress, geranium, juniper, lavender, patchouli
Dehydrated Skin	Chamomile, clary sage, lavender, rose otto
Acne	Cedarwood, chamomile, cypress, eucalyptus, juniper, lavender, patchouli, rosemary, tea tree, vetiver
Sensitive Skin	Try half per cent concentrations of chamomile, lavender, rose otto
Combination Skin	Geranium, lavender, neroli, rose otto
Thread Veins	Chamomile, cypress, lemon, rose otto

Foot and Hand Baths

These can be used to ward off chills as well as rheumatic or arthritic pain, excessive perspiration, athlete's foot and other skin disorders of the feet or hands such as dermatitis or eczema.

Sprinkle five-to-six drops of essential oil, diluted in vegetable oil if desired, in a bowl of hand-hot water and soak feet, or hands, for about ten minutes. Dry thoroughly and massage in a little vegetable oil, or cream, containing a few drops of the same essence(s).

Compresses

A compress is a valuable way of treating muscular pain, sprains and bruises as well as reducing pain and congestion in internal organs. However, it is vital to know when to apply a cold compress and when to apply a warm compress.

Cold: *These are for recent injuries such as sprains, bruises, swellings, inflammation and headaches.*

Warm: *These are for old injuries, muscular pain, toothache, menstrual cramp, cystitis, boils and abscesses.*

To make a warm compress, add about six drops of essential oil to a bowl of water containing about half a litre of water, as hot as you can comfortably bear. Place a small towel, or a piece of lint, or cotton fabric, on top of the water. Wring out the excess and place the fabric over the area to be treated. Cover this with a piece of clingfilm, then lightly bandage in place if necessary (for an ankle or knee for example). Leave the compress on until it has cooled to body temperature; renew at intervals as required.

For a cold compress, use exactly the same method as above, but with very cold, preferably icy, water. Leave in place until the compress warms to body heat, then renew at intervals as required.

Inhalations

Inhalations can help colds, influenza, sinusitis, coughs, catarrh, hay fever and other respiratory disorders. They can also be used to bolster a flagging memory. Essences of basil, rosemary and peppermint are known to have 'cephalic' properties – they stimulate clarity of thought. The simplest method is to put five-to-ten drops of essential oil on to a handkerchief and inhale as required. Drops of the appropriate essential oil can also be sprinkled on to your pillow to ease nasal congestion and to aid restful sleep. If you do not wish to put essential oils directly on to the pillow, put them on a clean handkerchief and leave nearby.

A more powerful decongestant is the steam inhalation – but avoid this if you suffer from asthma. Steam inhalations can be employed to help other respiratory problems such as those mentioned above, or as a deep cleansing facial (see page 41).

Pour about half a litre of near-boiling water into a bowl and then add two-to-four drops of essential oil. The quantity depends on the strength of the essence. Peppermint, for example, is extremely powerful, whereas sandalwood is very mild. Inhale the vapours for about five minutes, but no longer than ten. In order to trap the aromatic steam more efficiently, drape a towel over your head and the bowl to form a 'tent', as with the facial sauna.

You can enjoy steam inhalations two or three times a day over a short period, if you are suffering from a cold or influenza.

Using Undiluted Essential Oils
Provided the skin is cooled first under cold running water, eucalyptus, tea tree or lavender can be applied neat to burns and scalds. It can also be applied neat to cuts, grazes, wounds, insect bites and stings. Lavender is a particular favourite because it is less likely to irritate sensitive skin. Moreover, undiluted lavender essence is also remarkably effective for athlete's foot.

Perfuming Rooms
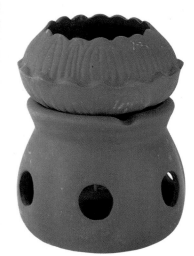
The best way to perfume a room is to use a purpose-designed essential oil burner/vaporiser, or an electric diffuser. These are now widely available from health shops and essential oil suppliers. A few drops is all you will need for at least an hour of fragrance. Follow the manufacturer's instructions for use. If you are not able to obtain either of these gadgets, see for other, although less effective, methods of perfuming rooms.

Put a drop or two on a damp pad of cotton wool or a handkerchief and place it on a radiator. Better still, add a few drops of essential oil to the water of a radiator humidifier. Another method is to put a couple of drops on a cold lightbulb so that when you switch on the light, the oil will vaporise into the room with the heat of the bulb. You may prefer to buy a moderately-priced fragrance ring. This is a ceramic or cardboard disc that balances on top of the lightbulb. The essences are dropped on the disc and the warmth from the bulb releases the aromatic vapour. Essential oils can also be vaporised in the molten wax of a burning candle. However, it is important to obtain a very fat candle which will produce a good-sized pool of wax around the wick, thus enabling the oil to vaporise slowly. First light the candle. Wait for the wax to melt, then blow it out and immediately add a few drops of essential oil around the wick before re-lighting. Essential oils are highly flammable, so if you attempt to add the oils while the candle is still burning, it will flare up, leaving a puff of black smoke in its wake. It is also important to keep the wick very short, otherwise the flame will be too high and the aromatic vapour short-lived.

Essential oils can also be used as fumigants to help prevent the spread of infection during epidemics. The following essences are the most powerful against air-borne bacteria: pine, thyme, peppermint, lavender, lemon, rosemary, clove, cinnamon, eucalyptus and tea tree. The last two oils are also credited with anti-viral properties as well, and are useful for combating influenza. Vaporizing equipment is the best way to fumigate a room, although a plant spray could be used instead. Add five drops to 145ml of water and shake well before use.

Of course, rooms perfumed with essential oils have a subtle effect on the mood of their occupants. Frankincense, for example, will enhance meditation or yoga practice; orange and clove will help bring a winter's party to life; lavender and neroli will soothe and aid restful sleep at the end of a hectic day.

Skin Perfumes

Essential oils can be used singly or blended with other essences to make delightful perfumes. They may be used purely for pleasure or to support the healing action of other aromatherapy treatments. This is particularly true of stress-related problems. For the occasional anxiety attack or depression, a blend of carefully selected essences will uplift the spirits. However, if anxiety or depression become a way of life, it is advisable to seek the help of a professional counsellor, aromatherapist or other holistic practitioner.

The blending hints that follow will not only help in the creation of wonderful skin perfumes, but also in the blending of massage oils and other aromatic concoctions (see also the 'Aromatic Concoctions' section in Chapter 7).

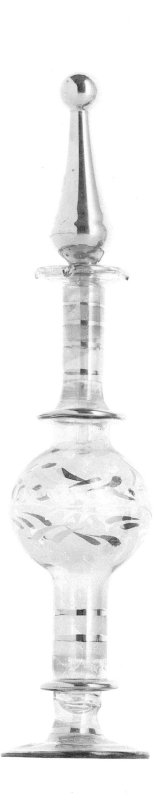

Creative Blending

There are no rigid rules about blending, at least as far as aromatherapy is concerned – although perfumers may disagree. It is purely a matter of how an aroma makes you feel, what it makes you think of? And is it a feeling or thought you would like to have more often?

Of course, there is no reason why you should not use a single essential oil if you are intrigued by its aroma. Rose, sandalwood and ylang-ylang are popular used singly, although aromatherapists often feel they work better when blended with other essences.

In simple terms, a 'well balanced' perfume is composed of top, middle and base notes, just as in music. The top notes of a blend are highly volatile – and do not last very long. These are essences such as bergamot, lemon and coriander. They form the scent's first impression, giving brightness and clarity to the blend, much as a flute adds high-pitched purity to an orchestra. The middle or 'heart' notes last a little longer, imparting warmth and fullness to the overall fragrance. Rose otto, geranium and ylang-ylang are some of the most popular middle notes. Then there are the heavier-smelling, deeply resonating base notes which profoundly influence the blend: patchouli, vetiver and sandalwood. They last a long time and 'fix' other essences. This means that they slow down the volatility rate of the top and middle notes, thus improving on the staying power of the blend, whether it be a skin perfume or a massage oil mix.

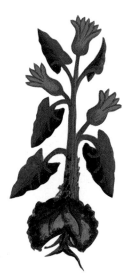

This musical analogy can help in making lovely aromatic blends if you are artistically adventurous. Indeed, anyone with a little flair can concoct pleasant aromatherapeutic blends once they become confident enough to experiment. If you are totally perplexed about blending, however, remember that 'families' of essences generally blend harmoniously: herbs (basil, clary sage, lavender, marjoram, rosemary), citrus (bergamot, grapefruit, lemon, orange), flowers (rose, ylang-ylang). Other compatible blends are spices with citrus (coriander and ginger with bergamot) and blends of woody essences (sandalwood with juniper, cypress or pine). Woods and resins are a good match too: frankincense with cedarwood is a classic. But why not be more adventurous? Try blending totally unrelated essences such as frankincense with rose or lavender; neroli with clary sage; sandalwood with lemon and ylang-ylang.

Even though perfumers may use numerous ingredients to create their sophisticated formulas, aromatherapy blends rarely contain more than three-to-five essences. Unless skilfully blended, the aroma can become rather 'murky' if more than a few essences are mixed together. The exception to this 'less is best' rule can be seen in eau-de-Cologne blends which contain a number of citrus essences. It is because citrus oils are so similar to each other that they blend harmoniously, becoming almost as one. However, citrus essences resonate from the top, so a delicious eau-de-Cologne blend can never be more than a brief encounter.

By blending different essential oils, we not only improve the aroma of a single essence, but, more interestingly, we can control the effect of the oil on the mind and body as a whole. For instance, you may be feeling depressed and lethargic, yet love the gentle relaxing aroma of sandalwood. However, you may benefit from a more stimulating or uplifting aroma. This could be achieved by blending the sandalwood with a little bergamot, lavender, geranium, or pine, depending on your aroma preference (see the perfume notes chart overleaf).

Alternatively, you may be suffering from the kind of depression that results in anxiety and insomnia as well as aching muscles, a very common symptom. Therefore, you will need a muscle relaxant (see the therapeutic charts in Chapter 7), sedative, anti-depressant blend such as chamomile and lavender. To cheer this up a little or to add an interesting note, you could add a touch of ylang-ylang, bergamot or perhaps frankincense.

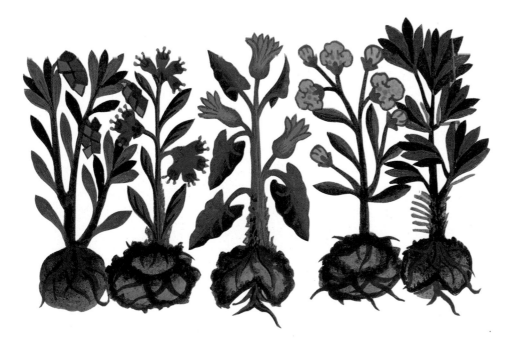

The Perfume Notes of Essential Oils

The following chart categorizes essential oils according to their perfume 'notes'. So, if you are determined to blend according to the rules, this will serve as a guide. Also included is the generally accepted psycho-therapeutic influence of each oil. However, we need to keep an open mind about this because people can respond differently to each essence, especially if they dislike the aroma.

Key: ✳ **(Top Note)**   ● **(Middle Note)**   ✚ **(Base Note)**

INFLUENCE	ESSENTIAL OIL	NOTE
Relaxing	Chamomile	●
	Clary sage	●
	Cedarwood	✚
	Cypress	●
	Juniper	●
	Marjoram	●
	Myrrh	●
	Neroli	●
	Rose otto	●
	Sandalwood	✚
	Vetiver	✚
	Ylang–ylang	●
Balancing *(stimulates or relaxes according to individual needs)*	Basil	✳
	Bergamot *(and all other citrus oils)*	✳
	Geranium	●
	Frankincense	✚
	Lavender	●
	Patchouli	✚
Stimulating	Black pepper	●
	Coriander	✳
	Eucalyptus	✳
	Ginger	●
	Peppermint	✳
	Pine	●
	Rosemary	●
	Tea tree	✳

INFLUENCE	ESSENTIAL OIL	NOTE
Anti-depressant	Basil	✳
	Bergamot *(and all other citrus oils)*	✳
	Chamomile	●
	Clary sage	●
	Frankincense	✚
	Geranium	●
	Lavender	●
	Neroli	●
	Patchouli	✚
	Petitgrain	✳
	Rose otto	●
	Sandalwood	✚
	Ylang-ylang	●
Aphrodisiac	Black pepper	●
	Cedarwood	✚
	Clary sage	●
	Coriander	✳
	Ginger	●
	Neroli	●
	Patchouli	✚
	Rose otto	●
	Sandalwood	✚
	Vetiver	✚
	Ylang-ylang	●
Anaphrodisiac *(a turn off!)*	Marjoram	●
Mental Stimulant *(for clarity of thought)*	Basil	✳
	Grapefruit *(and other citrus essences)*	✳
	Coriander	✳
	Eucalyptus	✳
	Peppermint	✳
	Rosemary	●

Prelude

Before going ahead and mixing a quantity of perfume, or any other aromatherapy blend, as directed in the recipe section (Chapter 7) you will need to find out whether the blend is compatible with your personality or present mood. There is nothing more disappointing than to discover that an enchanting-sounding blend is totally out of synch with your expectations. No doubt you will also wish to experiment with blends of your own devising, as suggested in this chapter. Here, then, are two methods for smell-testing your aromatic concoctions.

1. *Mix the sample combination of oils, up to six drops, in a teaspoon of vegetable oil. If you are intending to make a perfume rather than a massage oil, use the odourless jojoba oil as your base. Apply the blend to the inside of your wrist before smelling. The oils will then have the chance to interact with your skin chemistry. If you like the effect, dilute the blend to massage oil strength, as explained earlier, or develop the blend to perfume strength as outlined below.*

2. *To test aromatic waters and room perfumes, add up to six drops of essential oil to four teaspoons of warm water and mix well.*

CAUTION
The quantity of essential oil in skin perfume blends is quite high. If you have very sensitive skin or know that you have an allergy to perfume, you may have to forgo wearing even a natural perfume. However, you could perfume cotton outer garments with an aromatic water (see recipe section, pages 122–123) or enjoy room perfumes instead.

Perfume-making Procedures

Fill a 10ml dark-glass bottle almost to the top with jojoba oil. Build your perfume slowly, drop by drop, shaking the bottle after each addition and testing the smell as you go. You will need between fifteen and twenty drops altogether. Begin with the base note, if included, then develop the heart of the perfume and finally the top note. Once mixed, your perfume needs to be left for one or two weeks to mature. Keep it in a cool dark place, but remember to shake the bottle once a day to facilitate the process. At the end of the maturation period, the blend will have lost its 'raw' edge and will have an altogether more rounded aroma. If it seems too strong, dilute it with a little more jojoba.

In the next chapter we turn to the supreme application for aromatherapy – the art of massage.

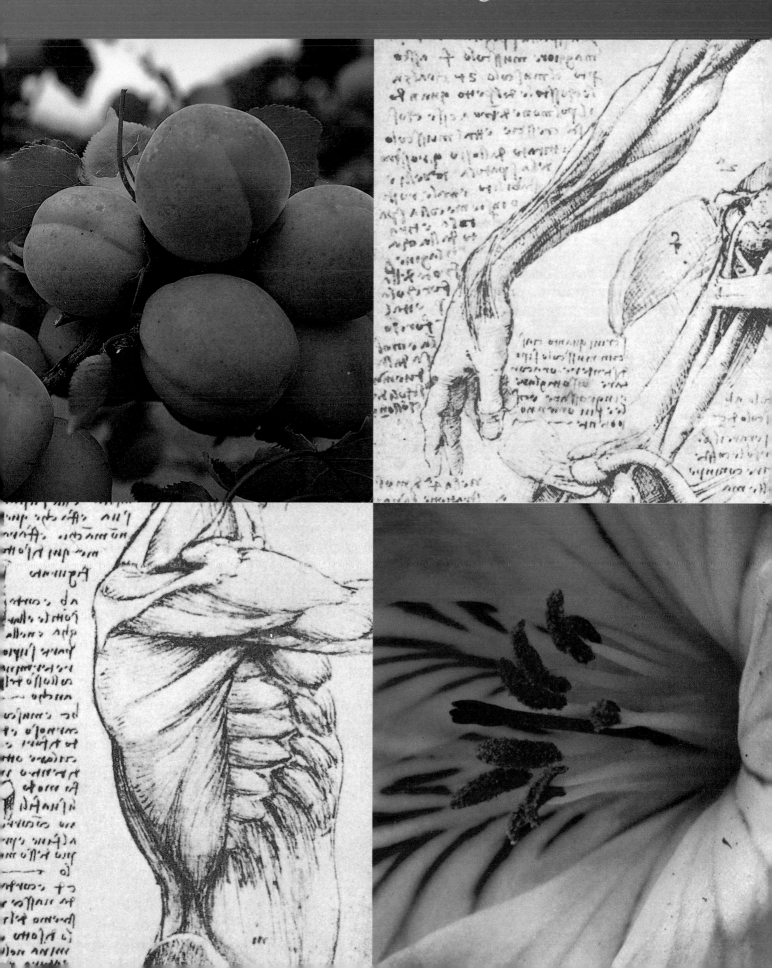

Therapeutic touch, be it the laying-on-of-hands or the more technical applications often associated with Eastern cultures, has always been part of healing the sick and the distressed. Indeed, while the East has a long tradition of massage therapy, the West is only now freeing itself from the idea that massage is just for tired sports stars or for clients of the 'massage parlour'. Few would have guessed, a decade ago, that aromatherapy massage would be playing a part in today's hospitals or be offered by family doctors.

The Effects of Massage

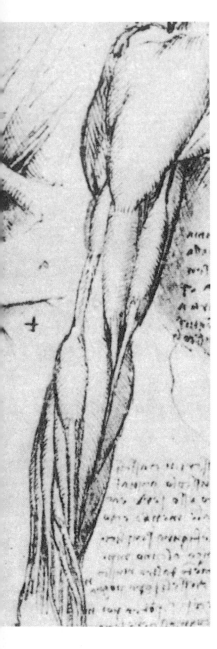

Physically, although massage cannot totally replace exercise, its effects are similar to twenty minutes' jogging – both stimulate the body. Regular massage, with or without essential oils, is especially beneficial to people who are forced to lead sedentary lives, perhaps through ill health, advanced age or physical disability. By improving blood circulation and lymphatic drainage, massage aids the elimination of tissue wastes such as lactic and carbonic acids, which often accumulate in the muscle fibres causing aches, pains and stiffness.

Equally, the emotional effects of skilled caring massage, especially if heightened by the aroma of essential oils, can be profound. Massage can create a peaceful, yet highly alert, state of mind similar to that experienced during meditation. As tense muscles begin to relax, pent-up emotions are also sometimes freed. Some people experience a light-headed sensation, as if they have had a few glasses of wine; a few fall deeply asleep; many become tranquil; others who are prone to tiredness and lethargy suddenly feel more alert and energetic. This is because massage exerts a balancing effect on the entire nervous system.

The Massage Giver

Unless an empathy is established between giver and receiver, nothing beneficial can come about. If you are giving massage you need to tune in to the needs of your partner, enabling you to sense which parts need soothing. With concentration, most of us can develop this sensitivity. If you follow the sequence described in this chapter, you will soon develop a good basic technique on which to build. One important point: when massaging talk as little as possible, give your attention to the movement of your hands and the feel of your partner's body so that a flowing rhythm can develop.

The Massage Recipient

If you are being massaged, you need to learn how to accept it passively and with full awareness; that is, by trusting your partner and opening up to the experience. If you constantly chatter and fidget, this is difficult to achieve. Instead, close your eyes, take a few deep breaths, then exhale with a sigh and relax into the experience. Focus your attention on your partner's touch and enjoy the sensation; allow your body to go heavy and limp. Do speak up, of course, if something hurts, or if you feel cold or uncomfortable. Also, if your neck starts to feel stiff when lying on your front, do turn it to the opposite side.

Setting the Scene

The room in which the massage is given should have a calm ambience and be very warm. Chilled muscles contract, causing a release of adrenalin, something you are trying to soothe away. Décor is important. According to colour therapists, jarring vibrations, emanating from zig-zag patterns or from vivid colour clashes, can affect us even when our eyes are closed. Neutral colours or pastel shades are far more conducive to relaxation. Massage in natural daylight if possible or under a soft lamp or candlelight. Harsh overhead lighting will remind you both of an operating theatre or a visit to the dentist! If you live in a noisy area, you may wish to block out background disturbance by playing relaxing music at low volume.

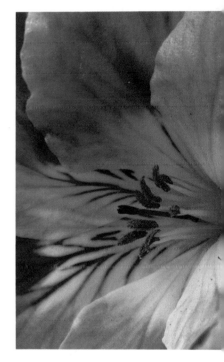

The Massage Surface

A purpose-built massage couch is ideal, but, in reality, it is more likely that you will have to massage at floor level. In fact, although this is hard work for the person giving the massage, it is better for the recipient because it will be easier for the giver of massage to apply beneficial pressure using their own body weight.

However, if you suffer from a weak back or poor muscle tone, giving massage on the floor will feel very uncomfortable and you will probably ache afterwards. It is important, therefore, to build up stamina and flexibility with a sensible exercise programme before massaging others. Gentle stretching exercises are beneficial, especially yoga.

A couple of sleeping bags, placed one on top of the other, a strip of foam rubber, thick blankets, a soft rug or a folded double-size duvet on the floor, will provide the necessary padding under your partner. If you must use a bed, ensure that the mattress is firm. If it is too soft, your partner will sink into it, and the mattress will absorb the pressure intended for your partner's body.

Whatever working surface you choose, cover this with a sheet or a large towel. To prevent your partner from getting cold, a second sheet or bath towel will be needed to cover areas of the body you are not working on.

CAUTION
When giving massage on a bed, or at floor level, never stand bending from the waist. Apart from impeding the all-important flow of the massage, this will put an enormous strain on the lower back. Get up onto the bed and kneel beside your partner. You should also kneel beside your partner if giving massage on the floor which should, ideally, be carpeted to protect your knees.

The Massage Oil

Essential oils are never used neat for massage; they must first be diluted in a good-quality vegetable oil (see Chapter 4). Do remember to take into account your partner's aroma preference, as well as their physical needs, perhaps offering a selection of 'possibles', then blending accordingly. You will need one- to one-and-a-half dessertspoons of oil for a full-body massage, perhaps more if your partner is very big and/or hairy, or has very dry skin. If you intend to massage only one part of the body, the face, feet or hands, for example, then you should need no more than one teaspoon of oil. Put the oil into an attractive dish and place nearby, taking care not to knock it over as you work.

When Not to Massage

It is unadvisable to massage if the recipient suffers from the following conditions: fever, inflammation (of skin or joints), thrombosis, advanced heart disease, phlebitis, varicose veins, skin ulcers, rashes or eruptions, swellings, bruises, sprains, torn muscles and ligaments, broken bones and burns.

In short, if something hurts, abandon the movement and move on to another area of the body. It is also generally believed, although recent evidence does not seem to bear this out, that people with cancer should not be massaged because cancer cells may start to spread to the rest of the body via the lymphatic system. Today, however, very gentle aromatherapy massage, without the use of percussion movements such as pummelling and hacking, is used in many hospitals and hospices to help lift the spirits of cancer patients.

About Aromatherapy Massage

The full-body massage sequence incorporates strokes used in traditional Swedish massage, a system developed in the early nineteenth century by Per Henrik Ling, the Swedish gymnast.

Ling chose French names, rather than Swedish, to identify the main massage strokes: effleurage (stroking), petrissage (kneading), tapotement (striking). The latter is not often used in aromatherapy, but for people who believe in the fallacy that massage must be vigorous if it is to do any good, I include these movements as an optional extra.

Aromatherapy massage is carried out much more slowly than traditional massage, and incorporates certain healing techniques borrowed from Eastern systems of therapeutic touch. The aim is to balance certain subtle energies (akin to electromagnetism) whose flow may have become impeded. An impeded flow of energy manifests itself as physical and emotional disharmony. A good massage can release a great deal of energy hitherto wasted in muscle tension, which is often, in itself, a reflection of emotional tension.

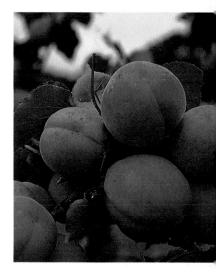

Massage Guidelines

Before giving massage, do ensure that your nails are short. No giver of massage should consider subjecting others to scratching and clawing!

Ideally, you will have an enthusiastic friend or partner with whom to exchange aromatherapy massage. By trying out the techniques on each other, you will develop a sense of how massage should feel. What feels good to you should also feel good to your partner. The following tips will help you to develop your own creative style.

1. *Keep the whole of your hands in contact with your partner's body.*
2. *When you need to apply more oil, try not to break contact with your partner's body. Keep one hand on his or her back, or arm, foot or head. Ideally, the whole massage should feel like a continuous flowing movement. A break in contact mid-flow can feel most disconcerting to the recipient. However, it is all right to break contact once you have reached a natural pause in the sequence, for example when you have finished working on the back of the body and wish your partner to turn over.*
3. *Add interest by varying the pressure from very light to very strong. It should be lighter over bony areas such as the shins and knees, but quite firm over large muscles such as those either side of the spine and the buttocks. Generally speaking, a firm touch feels good. Your*

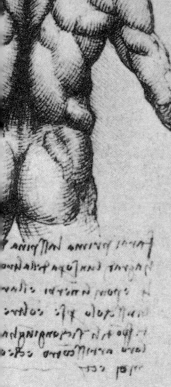

partner will tell you if you are applying too much pressure. Most beginners err on the side of too little pressure, which can feel ineffectual, or even worse, tickle intensely.

4. *Slow movements calm while brisk movements stimulate.*

5. *Try to work with your whole body, rather than just your hands and arms. When you are kneading, move gently from side to side in time with your hands. When applying pressure, lean into the stroke, using your body weight rather than overworking the muscles in your arms and wrists.*

6. *If you forget what to do next, simply stroke the skin with long gliding movements until you remember. It is far better to improvise than to stop mid-flow.*

7. *To give a good massage, you need to be totally relaxed and confident, otherwise your partner will sense your nervousness.*

8. *Do remember that sensitivity combined with the sheer pleasure of giving a massage, no matter how basic, far outweighs a full routine of complicated strokes carried out in a mechanical and impersonal manner.*

Timing

A full-body massage can take between one and one-and-a-half hours to complete. However, if you have only fifteen to twenty minutes to spare, it is better to give a shorter, quality massage to just one part of the body. The head, face, neck and shoulders; the hands or the feet; or a back massage, which includes the neck and shoulders, are good short-time areas. Moreover, while you are learning, it is easier to concentrate on just one part at a time – the prospect of doing a full-body massage can seem daunting at first.

Dealing with Muscle Tension

Once you become accustomed to the practice of massage, you will notice areas of the body that feel stiff, taut or even lumpy. Small nodules under the skin are caused by bunched-up muscle fibres and an accumulation of waste products. Sometimes these are so hard that beginners mistake them for bones! Soothe away any tension you find by stroking the surrounding area. Even more effective at easing out tension is the application of thumb pressure directly on to the taut or lumpy area (see page 101). Avoid, of course, causing any pain which will result in greater muscle tension. Be sensitive to your partner's responses and ease or deepen the pressure accordingly. It will help if you apply the pressure while your partner breathes out with a long sigh, and if you release the pressure as he or she inhales.

The Back of the Body

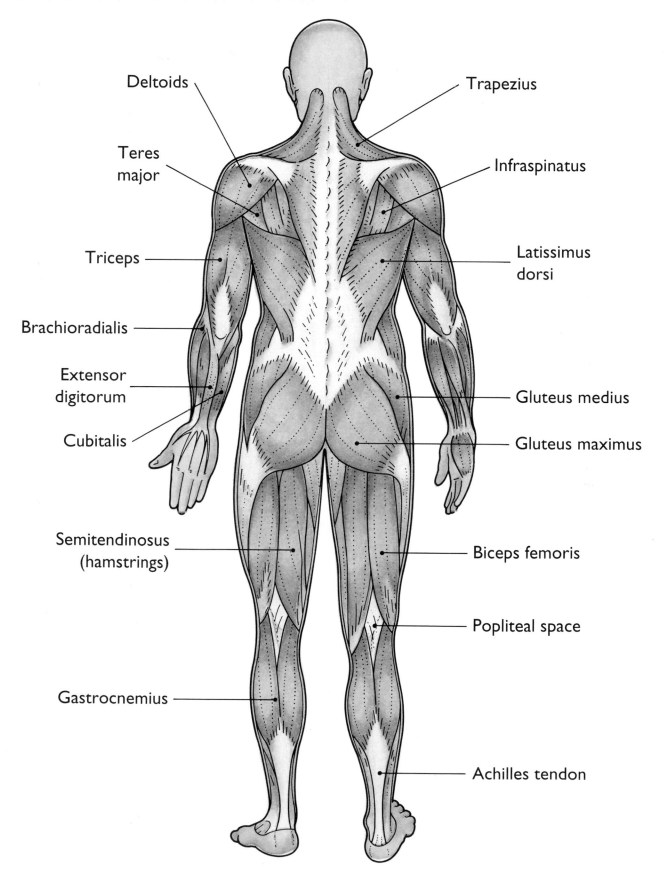

Deltoids

Teres
major

Triceps

Brachioradialis

Extensor
digitorum

Cubitalis

Semitendinosus
(hamstrings)

Gastrocnemius

Trapezius

Infraspinatus

Latissimus
dorsi

Gluteus medius

Gluteus maximus

Biceps femoris

Popliteal space

Achilles tendon

Massaging the Back of the Body

Ask your partner to lie on their front, head to one side, arms relaxed at the sides, or loosely bent with the hands at shoulder level. Some people feel more comfortable with a rolled-up towel or cushion under the chest and ankles. For warmth, cover your partner with one or two thick towels. If you are massaging on the floor, kneel with your knees slightly apart. If you are using a massage couch, stand with your feet slightly apart so that you are able to bend at the knees, enabling you to lean into the strokes.

Back, Neck, Shoulders and Buttocks

Since most massage strokes can be used on the back, this is a good place to begin learning the art of massage.

Never pour oil onto your partner's body – this can be quite a shock because the oil is usually much cooler than body temperature. Instead, oil your hands with the aromatic blend, using just enough to move smoothly over the skin without causing friction. When giving back massage on the floor, or on a firm bed, either kneel to one side of your partner or sit straddling their thighs – a very comfortable position which enables you to apply equal pressure with both hands.

Attunement
Before oiling your hands, place your right hand gently on the back of the neck. Place your left hand on the base of the spine. Breathe slowly and deeply, allowing yourself to relax. Hold this position for about half a minute. This will calm both of you and, at the same time, enable your partner to become accustomed to your touch.

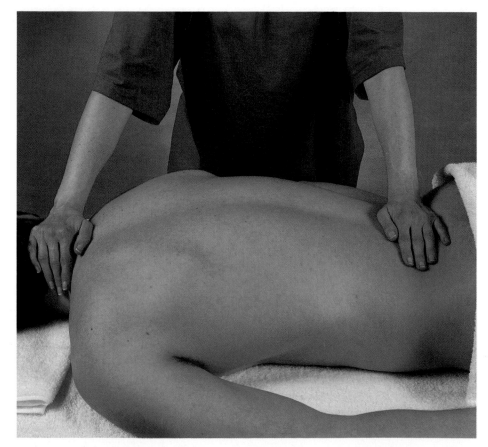

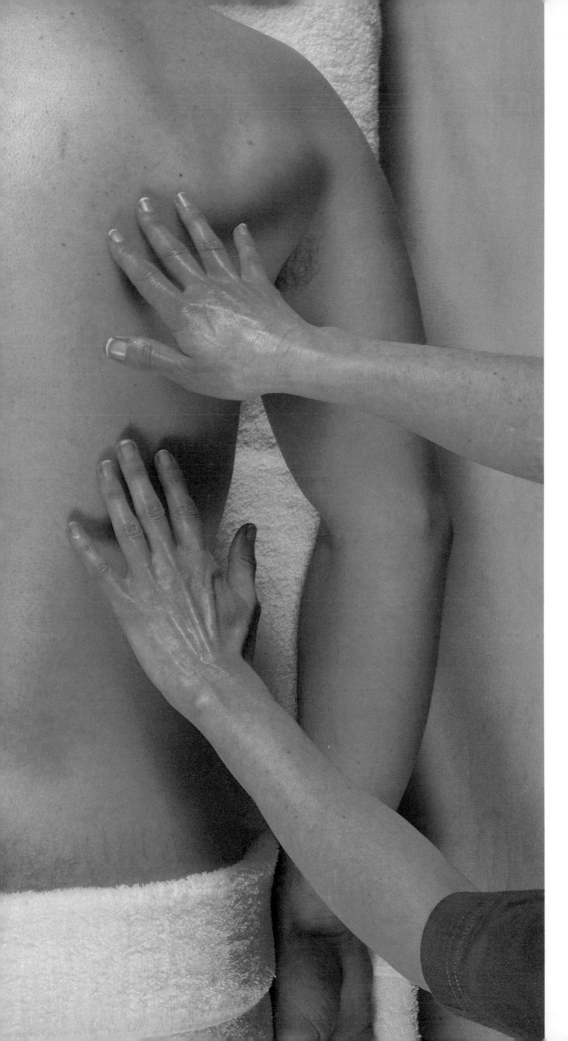

Feathering

Although not essential, the subtle technique of feathering – feather-weight sweeping strokes – is a wonderful way to begin or end a massage. Feathering may look superfluous, but it can have a profoundly soothing effect, especially if your partner is suffering from nervous tension.

Begin at the top of the head and move downwards over the whole body. With hands very relaxed, fingers loosely separated, feather-weight brush in one long sweeping movement down to the feet. The stroking should be, as the name implies, extremely light, barely perceptible to your partner. Take your hands back to the head and sweep downwards again. Do this at least a dozen times with rhythmic, flowing movements.

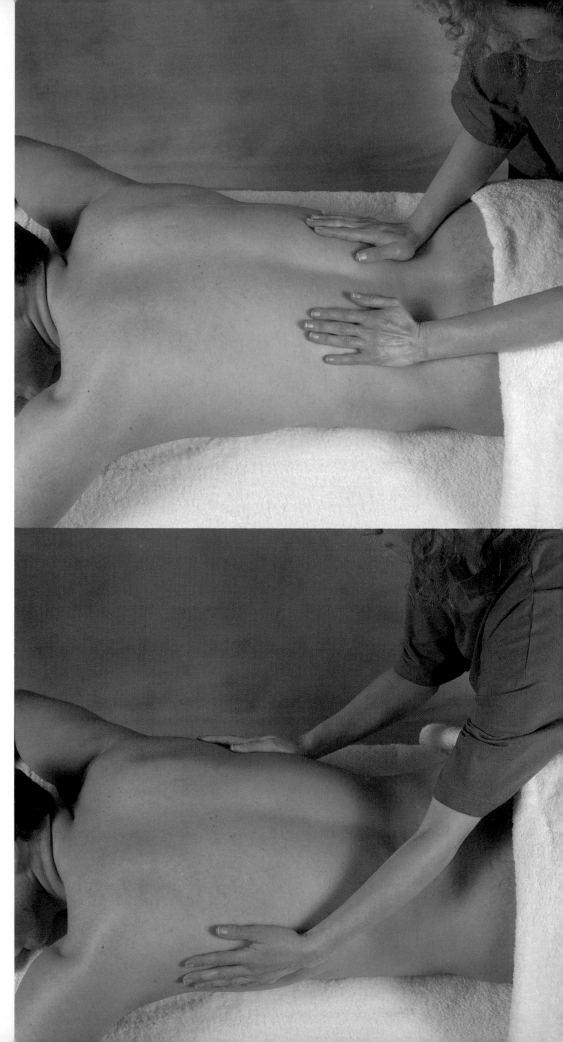

Gliding Strokes

1. *These transitional strokes are used on all parts of the body to begin and end a massage, and to ease the flow from one movement to another. Gliding is also the stroke used when applying oil.*

Place your hands at the base of the back, on either side of the spine, with your fingers relaxed, but close together, pointing towards the head. Never apply pressure to the spine itself, but to the strong muscles either side of the spine. Now glide your hands up the back until you reach the neck. Fan out your hands firmly across the shoulders, then glide them down. When you reach the waist, pull up gently and return smoothly to the starting point. Repeat several times.

60

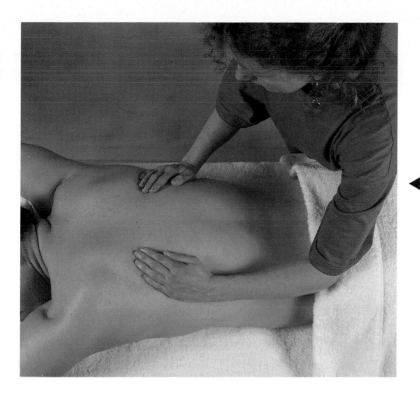

2. *As a slight variation, glide up the back, starting with your hands on the lower back as before, then glide firmly upwards. When you reach the shoulders, move your hands in circles over the shoulder blades. Then continue to make connected circles down the back, until you reach the* ◀ *starting position. Repeat several times.*

3. *The main strokes on the back can be done in either direction. The following back glide can be performed after the previous strokes or be used as an alternative movement.*

Position yourself above your partner's head. Place your hands on either side of the spine on the topmost part of the back, fingers pointing downwards. Glide your hands down the entire length of the back, to the tops of the buttocks, then fan out your hands over the hips and slowly pull them up the sides of the body. When you reach the armpits, fan out your hands over the shoulders then pivot them, turning the fingers towards the spine, so that they are back in the starting position. Repeat this movement several times. ▶

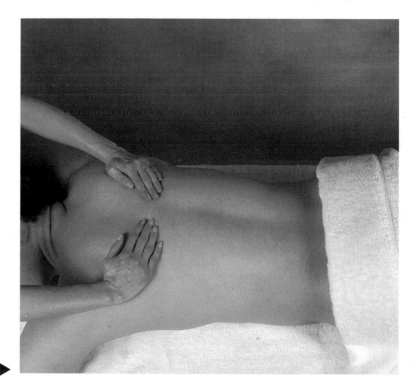

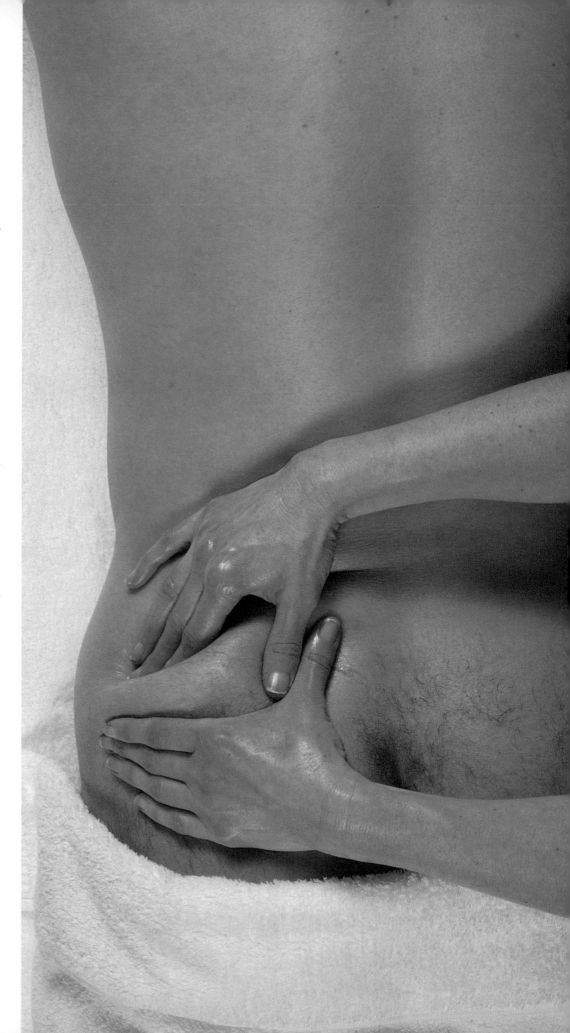

Kneading

Following on from the gliding strokes, kneading is carried out on the fleshy or muscular parts of the body. It consists of alternately squeezing and releasing handfuls of flesh in a broad circular motion. The purpose is to relax the muscles by draining away waste products and aiding venous and lymphatic circulation.

Using the whole of your hands, alternately grasp and squeeze the flesh (but do not pinch) as if kneading dough. Start at the hips and work up the sides of the body and across the upper arms and shoulders, paying special attention to areas of tightness (tension). Move to the other side of the body and repeat. The buttocks are often full of tension. Knead the first thoroughly, then move to the other. For more vigorous strokes – pummelling, hacking and cupping – see page 100.

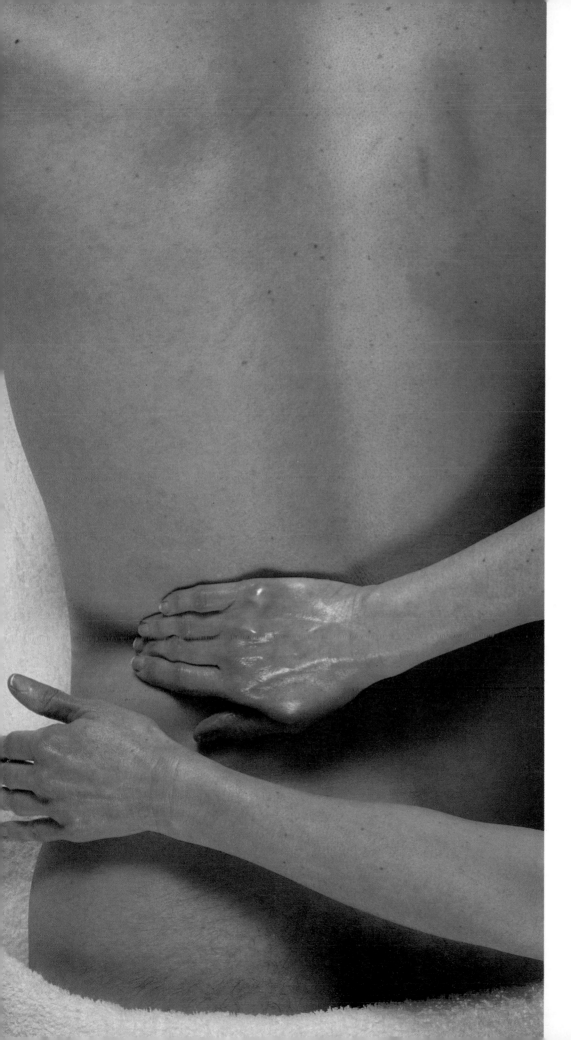

Pulling

This is a firm lifting stroke used on the sides of the torso and the limbs.

Move to one side of your partner's back. With your fingers pointing downwards, gently pull each hand alternately straight up, each time overlapping the place where the last hand was. Start at the hip and work your way slowly up to the armpit and back down again. Repeat on the other side.

Return to the long gliding strokes with which you began and repeat once or twice before moving on to the next stroke.

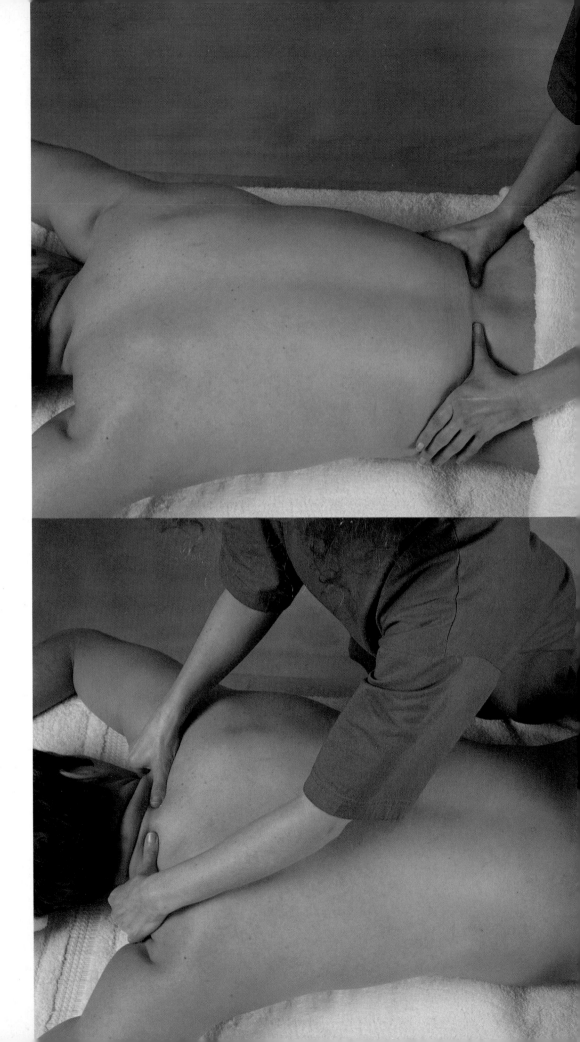

Friction

1. *The following movements make use of the thumbs or heels of the hand to reach deeper into the tissue to where hidden tensions lie. Only use friction after you have relaxed your partner's muscles with the previous strokes.*

This stroke for the lower back is similar to the gliding stroke, except that it incorporates thumb pressure. Position your hands, the thumbs pointing towards each other, as illustrated, either side of the spine. Keeping your whole hand in contact with your partner's body, lean into the stroke as you glide up the back to the neck. When you reach the top, fan out your hands across the shoulders, ease the pressure and slide them back down to the starting position. Repeat two or three times.

64

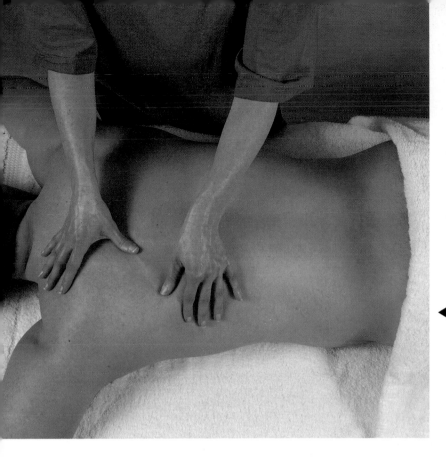

2. *Starting from the base of the spine, make small circular movements with your thumbs into the muscles either side of the spine until you reach the neck. With your thumbs on the upper back, continue the circular movements. Do not press on the spine or the shoulder blade itself. Work on the muscles just above the shoulder blades and those lying between them and the spine.*

Return to the gliding stroke and repeat two or three times before
◀ *moving on to the next stroke.*

3. *Apply some fairly strong pressure to the lower back by placing one hand over the other and circling with the heel of the hand. Using your thumbs as before, work on any areas of tension you may find there. Continue with several gliding strokes up the entire back before moving on to the neck and shoulders.* ▶

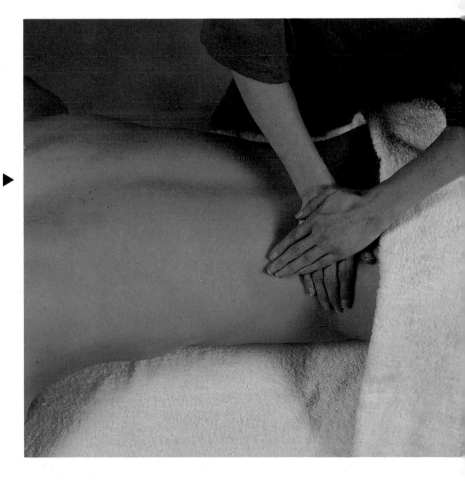

Kneading the Neck and Shoulders

1. *Ask your partner to move their hands to the top of the massage surface and rest their forehead on their own hands, as illustrated. Knead the neck muscles by working on both shoulders and up the neck to the base of the skull.*

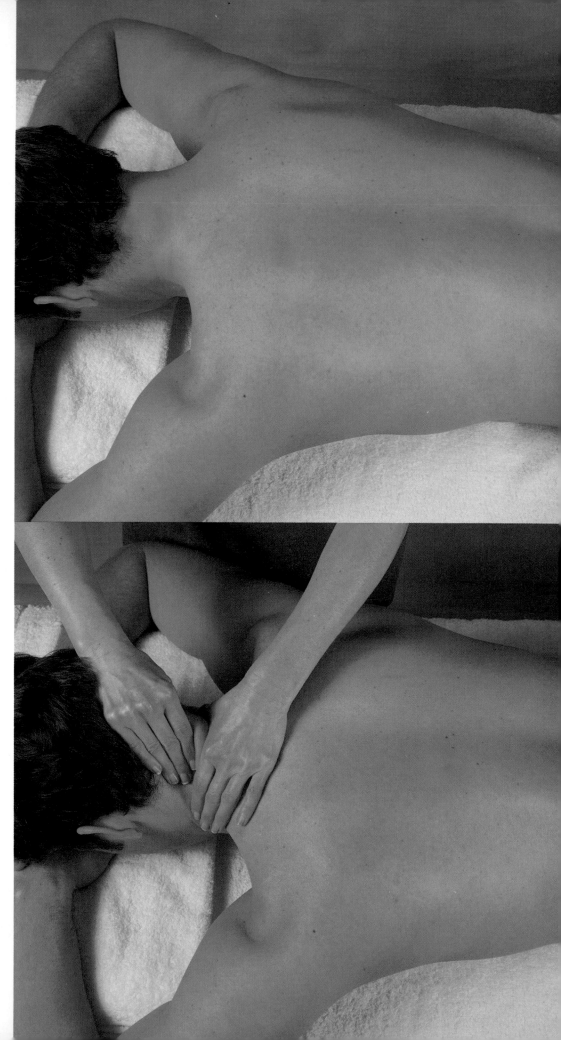

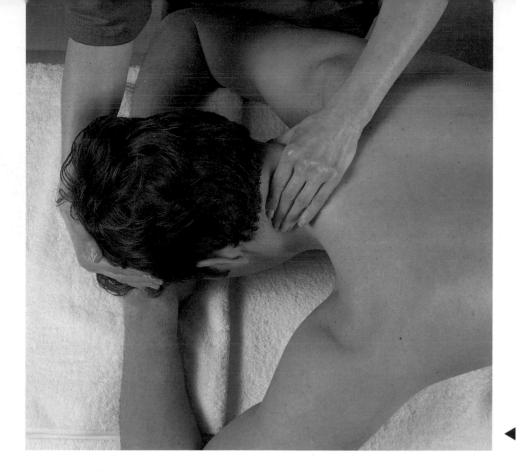

2. *Apply circular pressures either side of the neck, working up to the base of the skull. For this, use one hand, your thumb on one side and your index and middle fingers on the other. The other hand should be placed on the top of your partner's head to give a feeling of* ◀ *reassurance.*

3. *Ask your partner to release their hands and place their head to one side as before. Knead both shoulders at the same time.* ▶

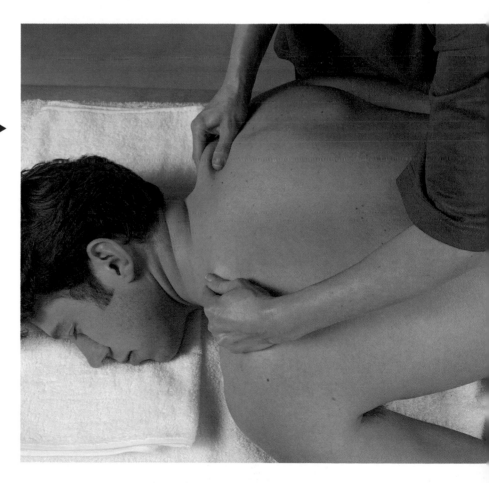

Working Under the Shoulder Blade

1. *Place your partner's hand in the middle of their back. Cup your hand under the shoulder joint and lift it an inch or two from the massage surface. This should raise the shoulder blade so you can begin working around and underneath it. Starting at the bottom of the shoulder blade, slide the edge of your hand slowly up and around the blade, pushing in under the rim. Repeat.* ▶

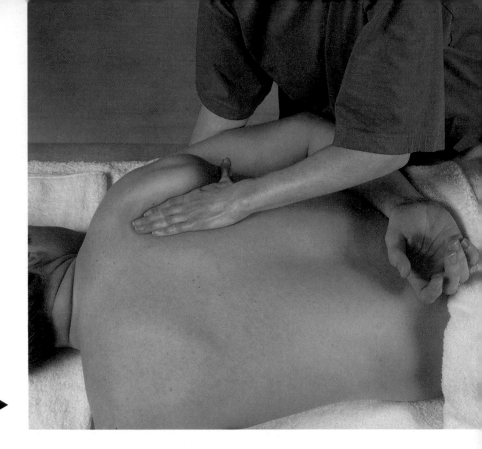

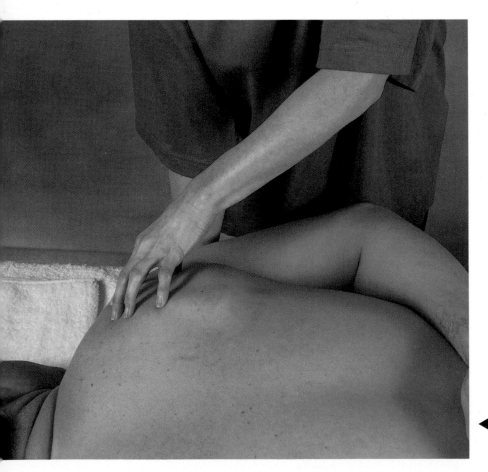

2. *To finish, shape your hand as if it were a claw, press firmly on the shoulder blade, and, using circular movements, slide the skin over the blade. Move several times to the right and left. Then move your partner's arm back on to the massage surface and repeat the same movements on the other shoulder blade.*

Return to the long gliding stroke and repeat two or three
◀ *times before moving on.*

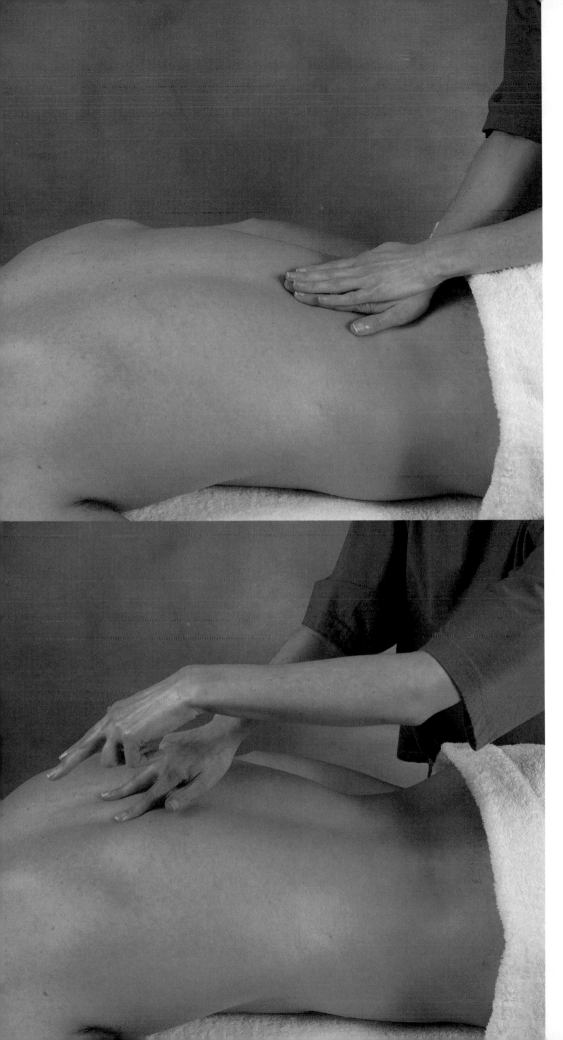

Riding the Waves

When done correctly, this stroke sends waves of relaxation up and down the spine. It is the only stroke that actually goes up the spine itself.

Place your right hand on your partner's spine, with the heel of your hand at the base, with fingers pointing towards the head. Place your left hand on top of the other hand as illustrated. Now slowly glide both hands straight up the spine, but do not press too hard. Using your index and middle fingertips press down firmly either side of the spine, with one hand overlapping the path of the other. Go all the way down to the lower end of the spine and off at the coccyx. Repeat once or twice.

Stretching the Back

1. *Starting from the middle of the back, place your hands side by side horizontally across the spine. Slide one hand smoothly but firmly to the right shoulder, and at the same time slide the other hand to the left hip, stretching the back. Repeat, taking the hands to the opposite hip and shoulder.* ▶

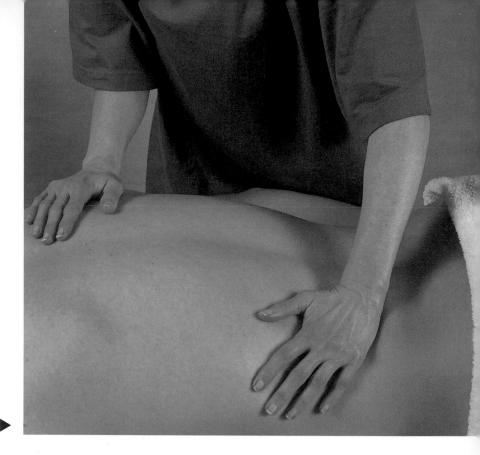

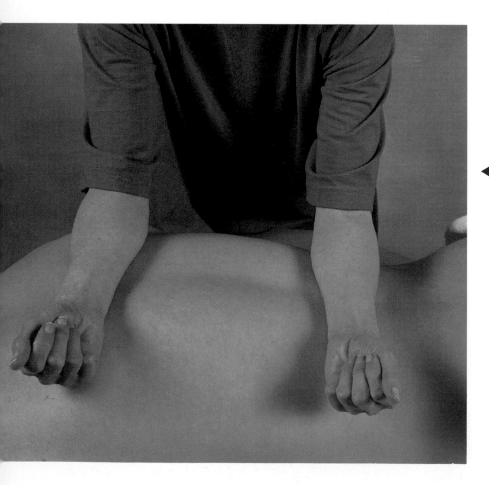

2. *Place the whole of your forearms horizontally apart across the back and slide them slowly, but firmly, one up the back to the top of the shoulders, the other down to the top of the buttocks, using* ◀ *a fair amount of pressure.*

Cover your partner's back with a towel. If you intend to finish your massage here, you might like to conclude with several full-body sweeps (feathering), as described on page 59. Having done that, place one hand at the base of the spine and one at the back of the neck and hold for about thirty seconds before moving quietly and slowly away.

If you are continuing, prepare to work on the legs.

Back of the Legs

1. Before applying oil, place your hands flat on the soles of your partner's feet and hold for several seconds.

▼

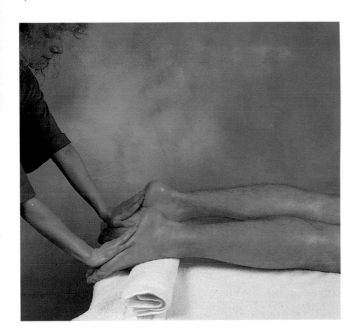

2. Oil your hands. Starting with the left leg, cross your hands over and, moving both hands together, stroke firmly up the leg from the ankle, going lightly over the back of the knee, to the start of the buttocks.

▼

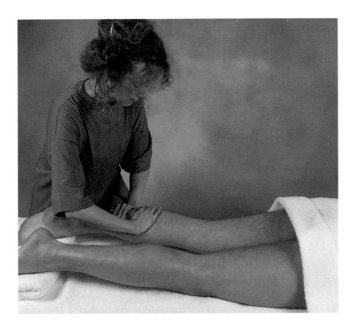

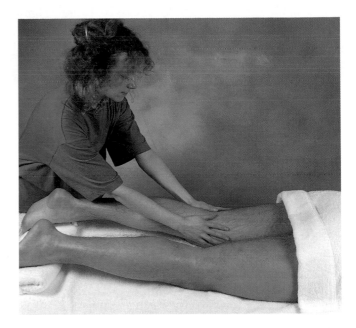

▲

3. When you reach the top of the leg, fan out your hands and, with a lighter stroke, glide down either side of the leg. Repeat several times, applying more oil as necessary.

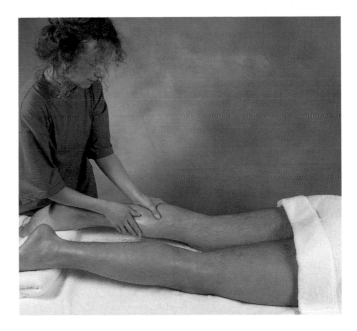

▲

4. Use your thumbs to apply friction to the calf muscles. Press firmly, moving your thumbs away from you in short alternating strokes all the way up to the start of the knee. The back of the knee is a very tender spot, so never apply pressure here.

71

5. *When you reach the thighs, press the heels of your hands alternately into the muscles of each thigh, using broad deep strokes.* ▶

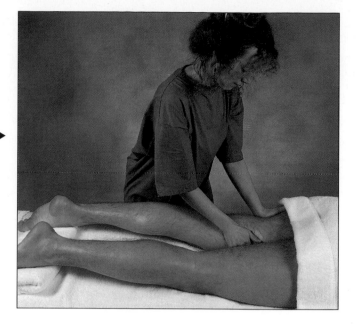

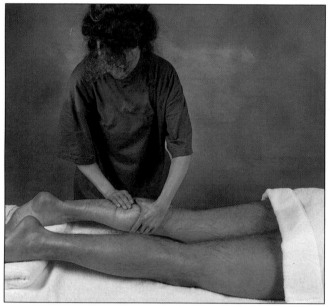

6. *Begin to knead the thigh, gently on the inner part, more strongly on the outer part where the muscles are larger.*

Knead the calf muscles with your two hands, using rhythmical ◀ *movements.*

7. *Bend the knee as far as it will comfortably go, and give a gentle bounce at the point of resistance.*

Return to the long gliding stroke and repeat once or twice. Cover the leg with a towel to keep it warm, then repeat the same sequence on the right leg. ▶

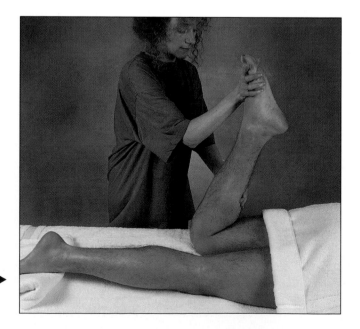

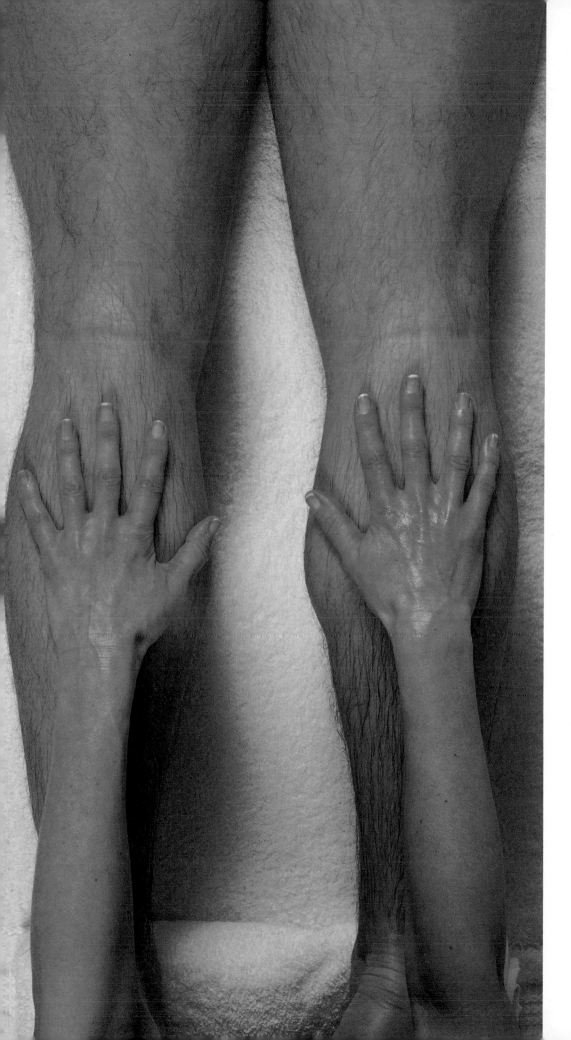

8. *When you have finished working on the right leg, remove the towel from the left leg and place your right hand, fingers pointing inwards, across the back of your partner's right ankle; and your left hand across the back of your partner's left ankle. Leaning into the stroke, glide up the legs to the start of the buttocks, fan out your hands and glide them lightly back down the sides of the legs to the ankles. Repeat once or twice before covering your partner's legs with a towel.*

Place your hands flat on the soles of the feet, as you did at the beginning of the leg sequence (see page 71), and hold for a few seconds before quietly asking your partner to turn over.

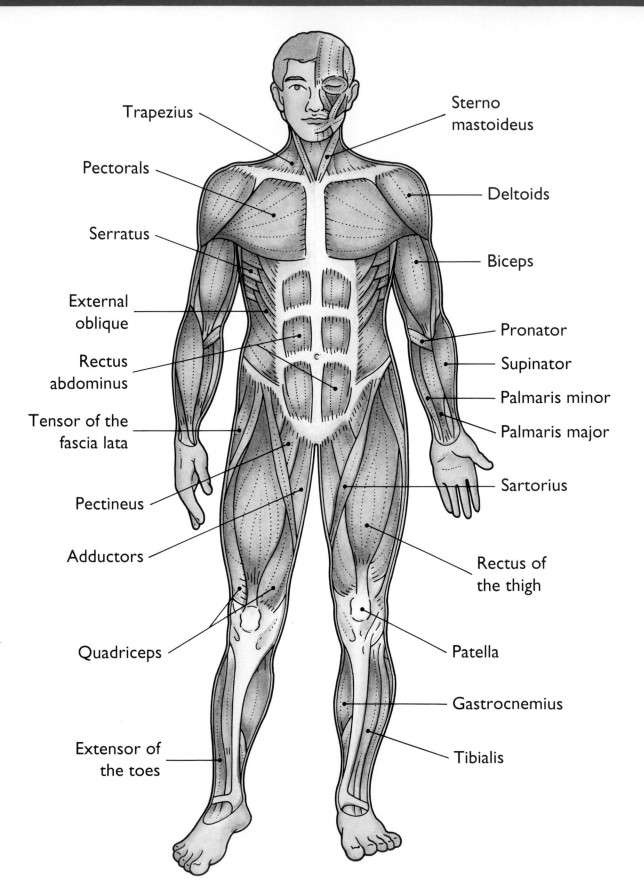

Trapezius

Sterno mastoideus

Pectorals

Deltoids

Serratus

Biceps

External oblique

Pronator

Supinator

Rectus abdominus

Palmaris minor

Palmaris major

Tensor of the fascia lata

Sartorius

Pectineus

Adductors

Rectus of the thigh

Quadriceps

Patella

Gastrocnemius

Extensor of the toes

Tibialis

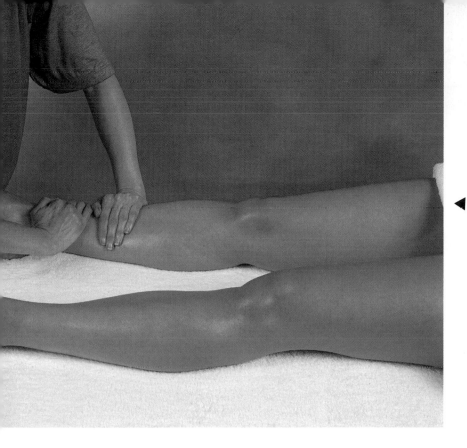

The Legs

1. *Oil your hands. Starting on the right leg, cup your hands over the ankle and stroke up the front of the leg. Do not apply direct pressure to the shin bone – this can be painful.* ◀

2. *When you reach the top of the thigh, fan your hands out and glide them lightly down the sides. Repeat several times.* ▶

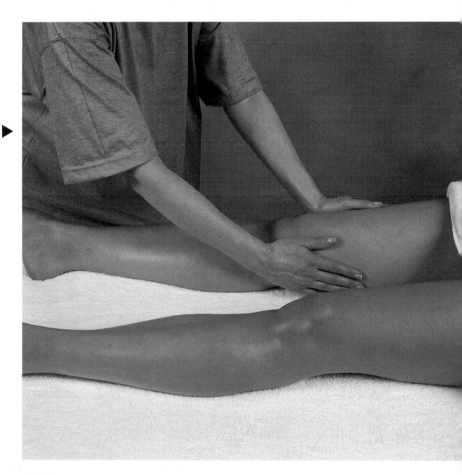

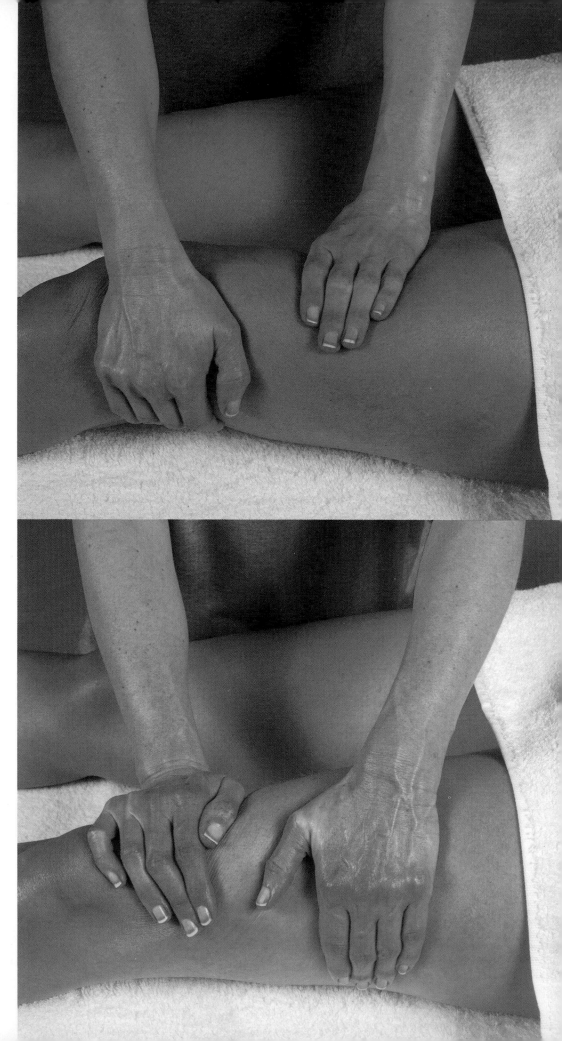

Push-and-pull Stroke

Return to the thigh and place your hands, fingers facing away from you, on either side. Now push firmly with your left hand and pull back with your right. Without stopping, change the position of your hands and push-and-pull in the opposite direction.

The Knee

1. *Start with your thumbs crossed just under the knee. Stroke up the sides of the knee to the top, one thumb on each side, allowing your thumbs to pass at the top.* ▼

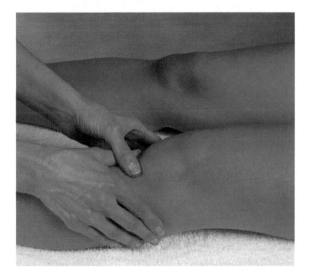

2. *Now stroke each thumb down the opposite side, both thumbs completing a full circle, passing the other at the tops and bottom. Repeat several times.* ▼

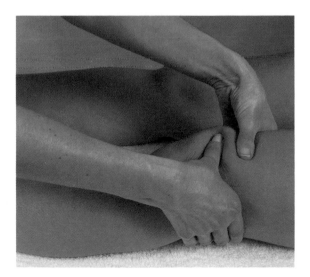

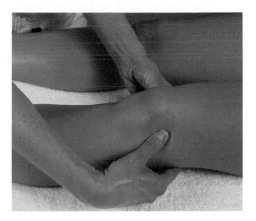

3. *Now use circular thumb pressures all round the knee, starting below the knee and working all around it.* ▲

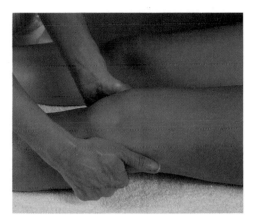

4. *Gently stroke the sides and the back of the knee with the fingers of both hands at once.* ▲

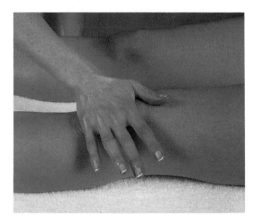

5. *Finish by rubbing the palm of your hand over the knee, gently rotating the kneecap.* ▲

Complete the sequence by stroking the entire leg from ankle to thigh.
Repeat the sequence on the other leg.

The Foot

The sole of the foot, and also the palm of the hand, contain thousands of nerve-endings with opposite ends located all over the rest of the body. So, massaging the feet or the hands stimulates other parts of the body, too. In fact, a good foot or hand massage has a balancing effect on both the body and mind, relaxing or stimulating according to individual needs. For this reason, when there is not enough time for a full-body massage, many massage therapists concentrate on a foot or hand massage.

As a matter of interest, the popular therapy known as reflexology uses special thumb pressures all over the foot (and sometimes the hand) to relieve tension and treat specific ailments. As the foot is believed to be a map of the whole body, reflexology is also used as a diagnostic tool. Pressure, applied to a specific reflex point, influences the organ or bodily system to which it corresponds. The lungs, for example, are reflected on the centre of the ball of the foot; the neck, all round the 'waist' of the big toe; the central nervous system, on the centre of the sole, just under the ball of the foot.

If there is a dysfunction in any bodily system or organ, crystalline deposits can be detected under the skin at the corresponding reflex point. The reflexologist works on these deposits in order to disperse them, thus activating the body's own self-healing mechanism. Some aromatherapists use reflexology as a diagnostic tool to determine which oils to use for individual clients.

It is beyond the scope of this book to teach the art of reflexology; the brief description given above is simply an interesting aside and an encouragement for further research.

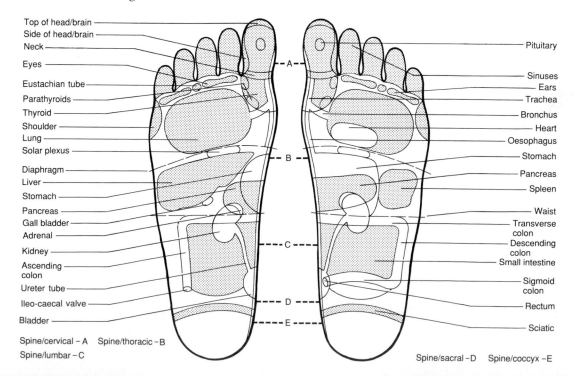

Top of head/brain
Side of head/brain
Neck
Eyes
Eustachian tube
Parathyroids
Thyroid
Shoulder
Lung
Solar plexus
Diaphragm
Liver
Stomach
Pancreas
Gall bladder
Adrenal
Kidney
Ascending colon
Ureter tube
Ileo-caecal valve
Bladder

Pituitary
Sinuses
Ears
Trachea
Bronchus
Heart
Oesophagus
Stomach
Pancreas
Spleen
Waist
Transverse colon
Descending colon
Small intestine
Sigmoid colon
Rectum
Sciatic

Spine/cervical – A   Spine/thoracic – B
Spine/lumbar – C

Spine/sacral – D   Spine/coccyx – E

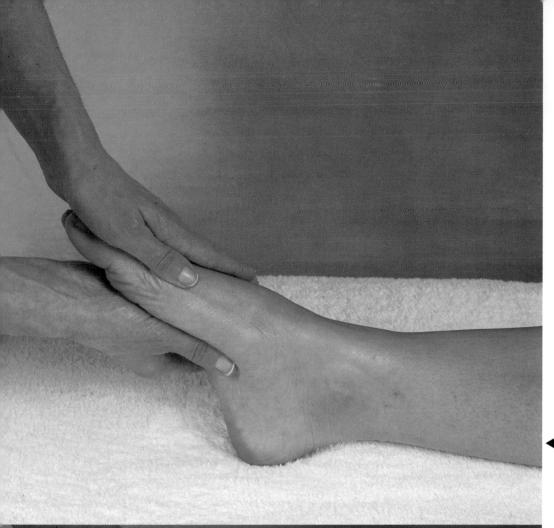

Foot Massage

1. *Unless the skin is exceptionally dry, the foot requires very little oil.*

Begin by stroking your partner's foot. Hold it between your hands and stroke firmly with both hands from the toes towards the body. When you reach the ankles, return your hands to the toes with a light stroke. ◀ *Repeat several times.*

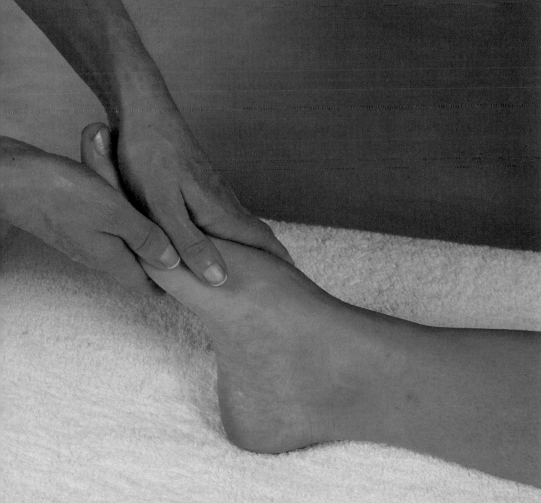

2. *Support the foot by placing your fingers underneath it with your thumbs on top at the base of the toes. Moving towards the ankle, make broad circles all over* ◀ *the top of the foot.*

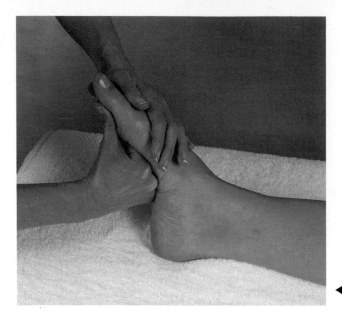

3. *Place your left hand across the top of the foot at the base of the toes. Make a loose fist with your right hand and position the knuckles just under the ball of your partner's foot. Gently manipulate the foot by pressing and rotating your left and right hands in a clockwise* ◀ *direction.*

4. *Work on the soles of the foot with the thumbs of both hands. Make small circles covering the entire sole.* ▶

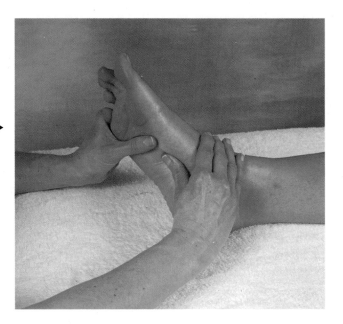

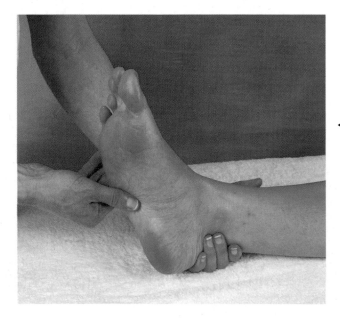

5. *Pinch the outer edge of the heels, continuing all the way up the outer edge of the foot to the* ◀ *little toe.*

6. *Now work on the toes. Starting with the big toe, gently squeeze and roll each toe between your thumb and index finger; rotate in both directions, then gently pull them towards you until your thumb and index finger slide off the tip of the toe.* ▶

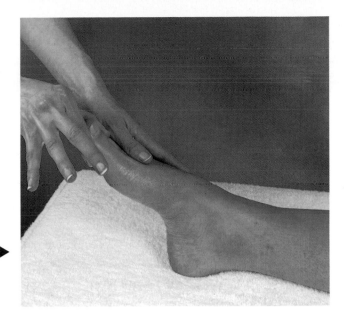

7. *Keeping one hand on top of the foot, bend your hand so you can massage the foot with the middle section of your fingers. Press firmly as you rotate your fingers, working* ◀ *all over the sole.*

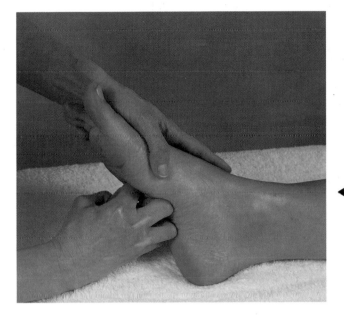

8. *Soothe the foot by stroking with the heel of your hand into the arch. Rest one hand on the top of the foot and stroke firmly down from the ball to the heel.* ▶

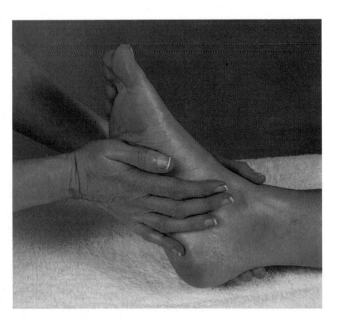

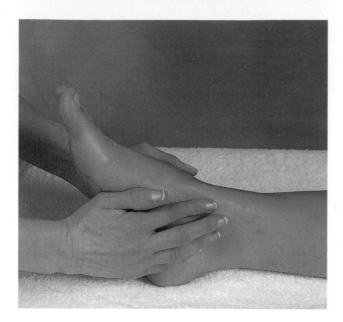

9. *Stroke the whole foot as you did at the beginning, then using your middle fingers with one hand on each side begin to apply circular pressures around the ankle.* ▲

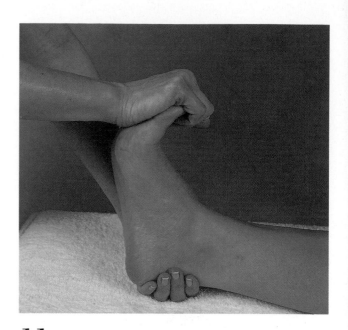

11. *To encourage flexibility, clasp all the toes with one hand and bend them gently backwards and forwards.* ▲

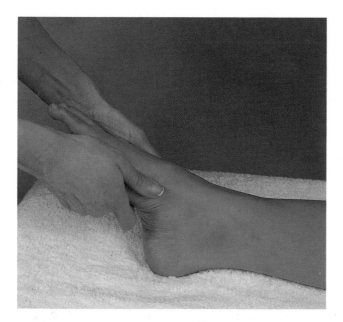

10. *Now stretch and squeeze the foot by grasping it with both hands, placing the heels of the hands against the top of the foot and pressing the fingertips into the middle of the sole. Using the heels of your hands, begin pressing firmly downwards on to the top of the foot. At the same time, very slowly let the heels of your hands slide from the middle out to either edge of the foot. Repeat two or three times.* ▲

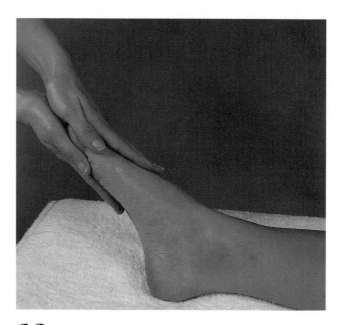

12. *Return to the stroking, with which you began, but this time slide your hands slowly off the end of the toes as illustrated. Repeat two or three times.*

Cover your partner's foot with a towel and repeat the entire sequence on the other foot. ▲

The Arms and Hands

1. Rest both your hands palms down on your partner's wrist and lower arm. Pressing firmly, glide both hands together up the arm. When you reach the top, separate your hands and glide them lightly back down the full length of the arm and over the hands. ◀ Repeat several times.

2. Using both hands, knead the forearm, working from the wrist to the elbow, then glide your hand down to start again. Repeat a ◀ few times.

83

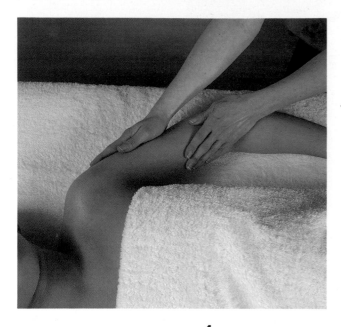

3. *Using both hands, stroke the upper arm from the elbow to the* ◀ *shoulder.*

4. *Knead the upper arm, from the elbow to the shoulder.* ▶

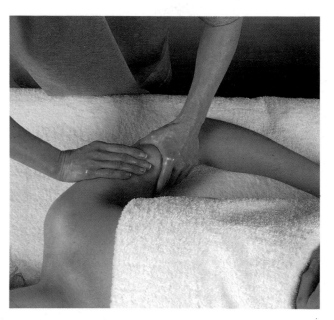

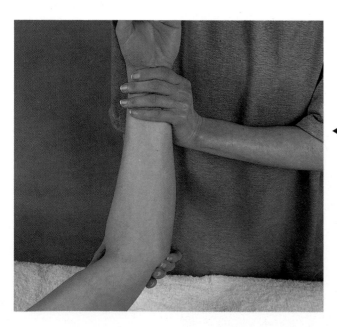

5. *Using plenty of oil (the skin here is usually very dry) massage the elbow by circling the elbow* ◀ *with your fingers.*

6. *Raise your partner's forearm, so that it rests upright, with the elbow supporting it on the massage surface. Then using the balls of your thumbs begin massaging the inside of the wrist. Use your thumbs, alternately as you work down the arm to the elbow. Repeat two or three times.*

Return to the gliding movement with which you began (see page 83), and repeat two or three times. ◀

7. *Finish the sequence with feathering. Using the fingertips of both hands, very lightly brush down the whole arm and off at your partner's fingertips. Repeat several times.*

Repeat the entire sequence on the other arm. ◀

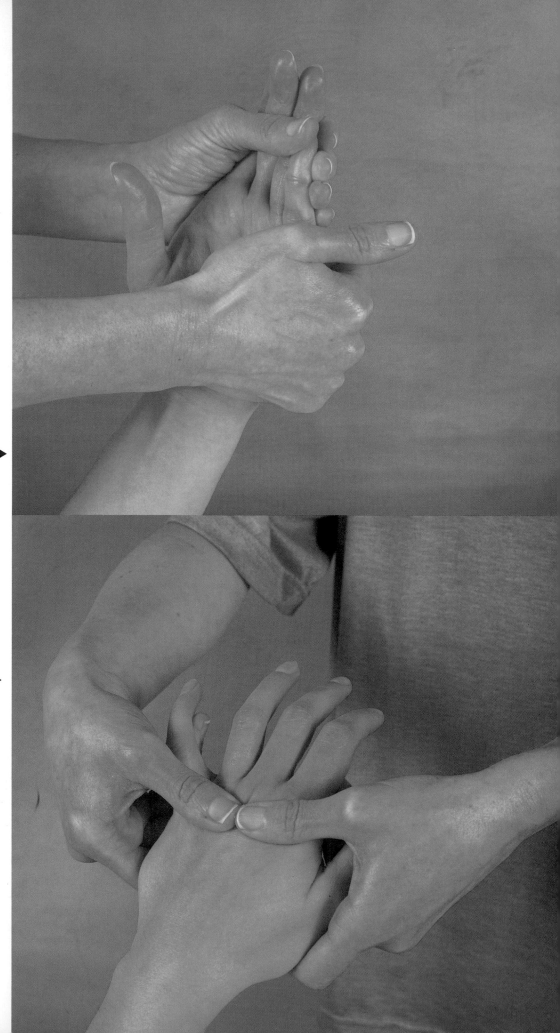

The Hand

The hand, like the foot, usually requires very little oil. Unless the skin is exceptionally dry, what is left on your hands after massaging the arm will be sufficient.

1. Using one hand, support your partner's hand, palm uppermost, and stroke the palm with the heel of your other hand, using firm, rotating movements. ▶

2. With both thumbs lying horizontally over the knuckles, press down and at the same time, flex the fingers towards you, giving the hand a good stretch. ▶

3. *Turn the palm uppermost, then, paying extra attention to the muscular area at the base of the thumb, firmly circle the thumbs all over the palm.* ▶

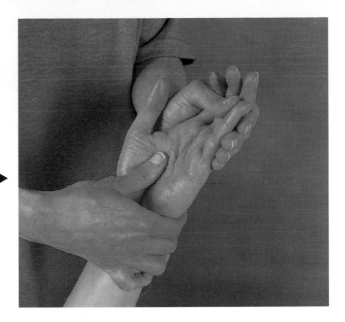

4. *Holding the hand palm-down in one hand and using the other to work on each finger, massage each finger. Paying particular attention to each joint, use circular thumb pressures along each finger, from the tip to* ◀ *the knuckle.*

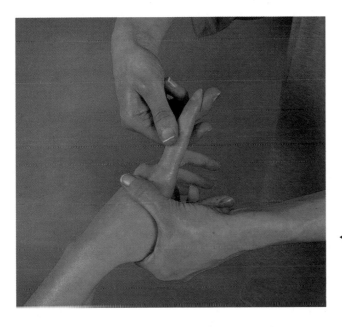

5. *Squeeze the outer edge of each finger, then gently pull them, giving a little twist as you slide your hand down and off the fingertips.* ▶

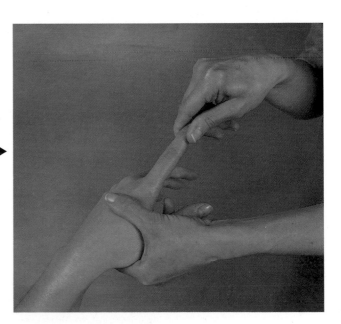

6. *Make a fist with one hand and place it on the palm of your partner's hand. Use the middle section of your fingers to make rippling rotary movements all over the palm.* ▶

7. *Stroke the whole hand, front and back, then sandwich your partner's hand between both of yours. Press them together firmly and hold for a few seconds. Release the pressure and slide your hands slowly off at the fingertips. Repeat a few times.* ▶

Repeat the entire sequence on the other hand.

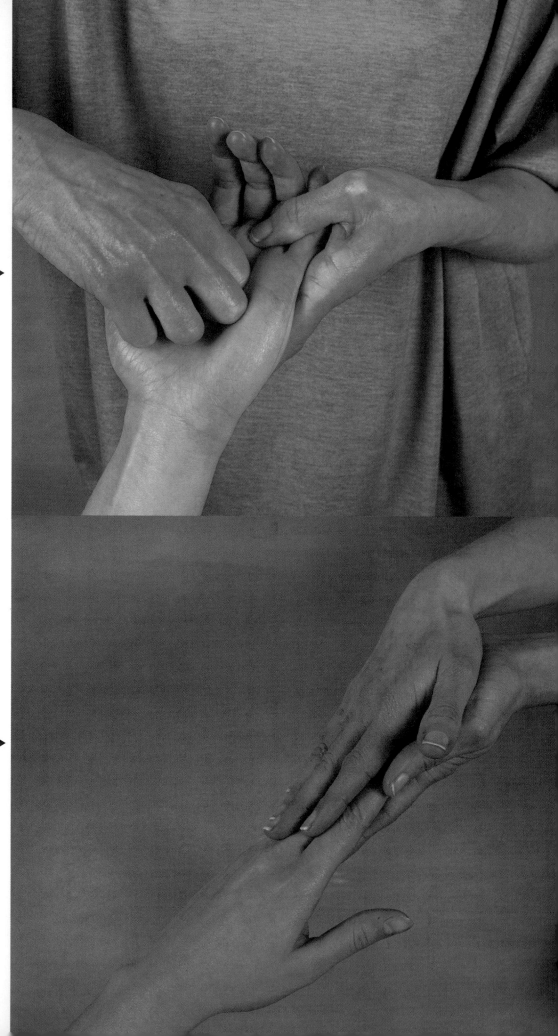

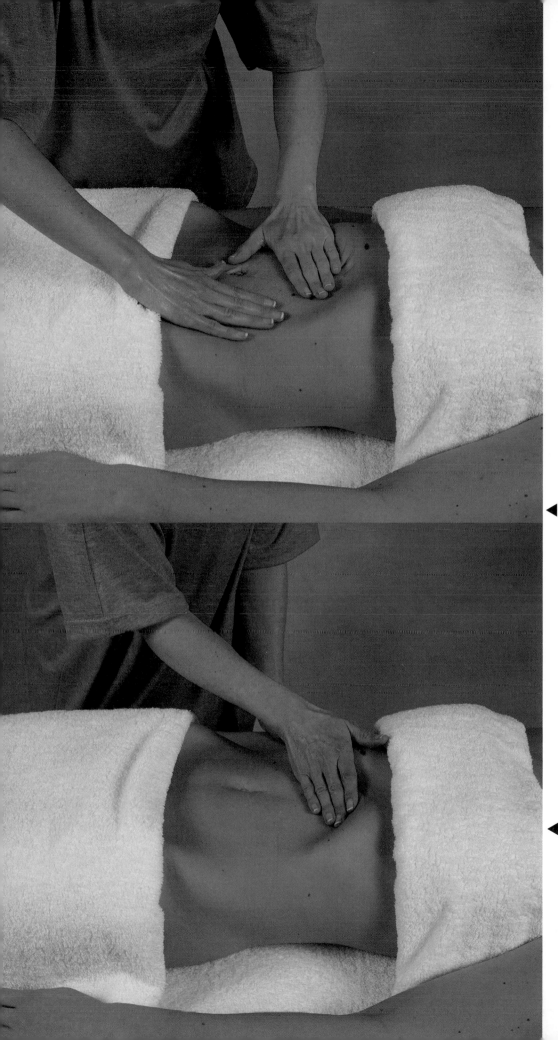

The Abdomen

Some people are apprehensive about having this sensitive area massaged. If your partner agrees, use only light pressure.

1. Move to one side of your partner; let your hands rest very gently over the navel for a few moments. Begin to massage the whole belly lightly, moving both hands (fingers and palms) clockwise around it, following the coil of the colon. You will find that one hand can complete full circles, but the other will have to break ◀ contact each time the hands cross.

2. If your partner is suffering from nervous tension, massage the midriff in an anti-clockwise direction. Using the right hand and resting the left hand on your partner's arm, gently stroke around the area several times before coming to rest over ◀ the navel.

Remember to cover your partner with a towel before moving on to the next stage.

The Face, Head, Neck and Shoulders

If your partner wears contact lenses, ensure that they are removed before you begin. The same applies to earrings, necklaces, or anything that might impede the massage. A good face, head, neck and shoulder massage can ease away tension headaches like magic! At the same time, by improving the circulation, it gives a healthy glow to the complexion. Only the lightest, fingertip pressure is required for the face, and it is important not to drag the skin. Use firm pressure over the scalp.

1. *Before oiling your hands, place them on either side of your partner's head, the heels of the hands covering the forehead and the fingers extending downwards, anchoring the sides of the head. Hold them there for a few moments.* ▶

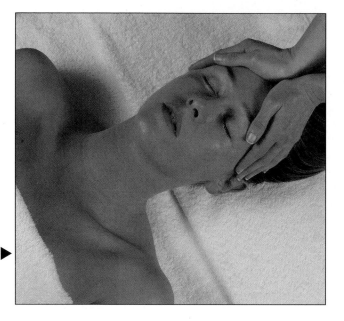

2. *Then move your hands to the forehead and smoothly stroke the brow, hand-over-hand, up and over the hair to the crown of the head.* ▶

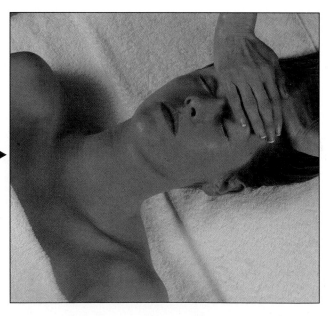

3. *Move your hands gently away, and oil them. Start with your hands lying next to each other, horizontally across the area just below the collar-bones, tips of the fingers touching, as illustrated.* ▶

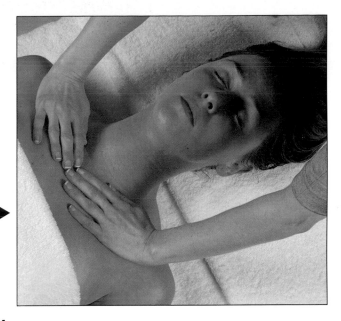

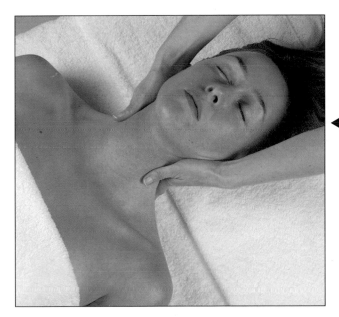

4. *Then slide your hands apart, moving across the top of the shoulders and up the back of the neck.* ◀ *Repeat a few times.*

5. *Cup your hands round both shoulders and gently push them down towards the feet to give the shoulders a good stretch. First push both hands down together, then alternately.* ▶

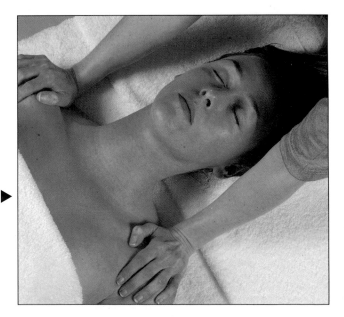

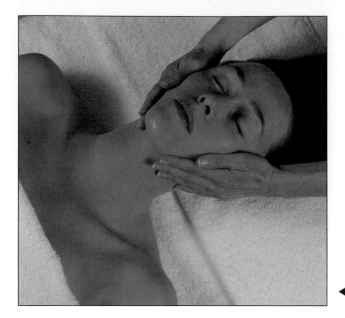

6. *Gently starting from the throat and sweeping up to the chin, use the whole surface of your hands, and slide your hands over your partner's face. Circle the cheeks, moving around the eyes (but not close enough for oil to seep in) and over the forehead. This is to oil the skin before you begin the main part of the* ◀ *massage.*

7. *Place the ball of your thumbs at the centre of the forehead between the eyebrows. Slide both thumbs apart and, when you reach the temples, finish with a little circular flourish before gliding off at the hairline. Return to the starting position, but this time a little higher up. Continue to stroke the forehead, a strip at a time, all the way up to the hairline.* ▶

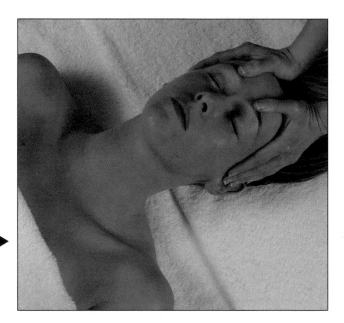

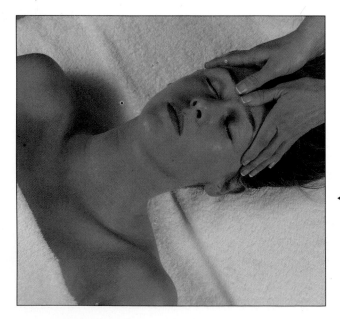

8. *Place your thumbs at the centre between the eyebrows (the 'third eye') and, this time, slide your thumbs a little more firmly over and beyond the brow bone. Repeat once or* ◀ *twice.*

9. *Return to the third-eye position and, this time, press your thumbs down quite firmly (your partner will tell you if it is too firm) and hold for about three seconds. Lift your thumbs and place them a little further out along the brow bone and repeat the pressure. Repeat this at intervals until you reach the outer corners of the eyes.* ▶

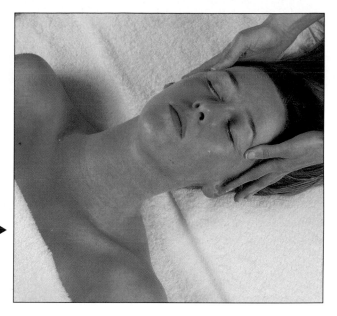

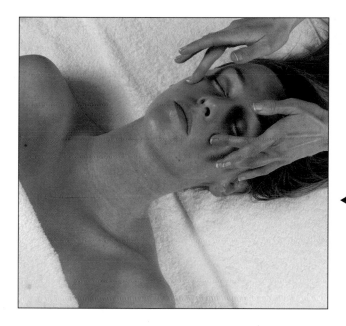

10. *Place your middle finger on the bony ridge under the eyes at the inner corners and repeat the pressing movements, a little more lightly this time, until you reach the outer corner. This is helpful for people who suffer from catarrh or* ◀ *sinus congestion.*

CAUTION: *Do not apply pressure if the sinuses are swollen and painful.*

11. *Allow your partner to bathe in darkness for a few moments. Place the heels of your hands gently against both eyes with the fingers extending downwards. Hold them there for no less than ten seconds. Gently stroke the entire face, neck and tops of the shoulders as you did at the beginning (see page 90), before moving on.* ▶

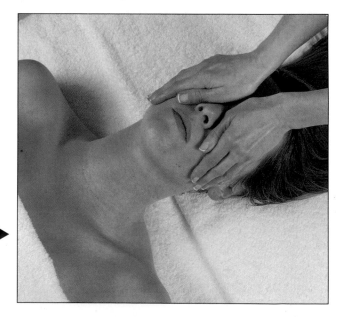

12. *Place the ball of your thumbs at the inner corners of the eyes just below the eye socket. Smooth lightly outwards and upwards towards the temples. Repeat a little lower down, a strip at a time, until you reach the edge of the cheekbone. Repeat the same movement again just below the bone, pressing lightly upwards.* ▶

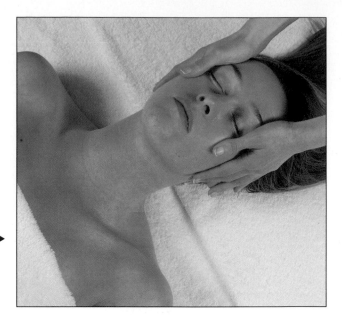

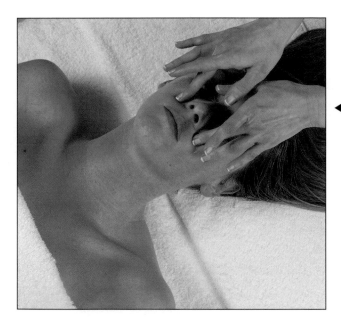

13. *Place the middle fingers on each side of the nose near the bridge. Using tiny circles, work down the sides of the nose.*

14. *Using your thumbs alternately, stroke down the bridge of the nose from the top to the tip. Circle the tip with the palm of your hand.* ▶

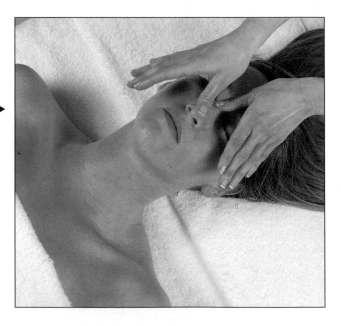

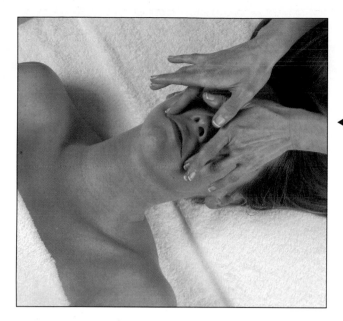

15. *Using your middle fingers, make tiny circles on the cheeks at either side of the nostrils and* ◀ *over the upper lip.*

16. *Place your thumbs on the chin and pull them slowly and firmly outwards and upwards along the jaw bone to the ear. Repeat a little further inwards until just below the cheek bone.*

Return to the chin and work in tiny circles with your thumbs, working from the middle of the chin along the jaw bone, finishing behind the ears. ▶

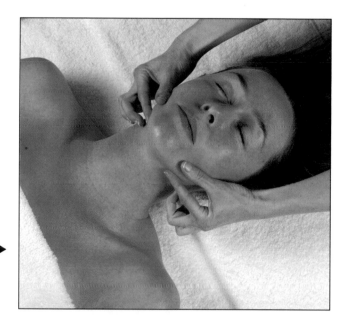

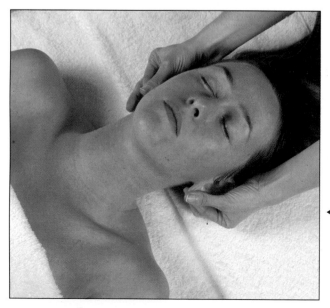

17. *Gently pinch the edges of each ear at the same time, from the top down to the ear lobes. Repeat once or twice, and finish by pulling the lobes gently downwards several times. Then with the tips of the forefingers trace around the spiral of the ears.*

◀ *Place the palms of your hands over your partner's eyes for several seconds before moving on to the neck.*

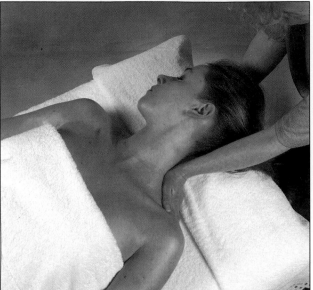

The Neck

1. *Oil your hands if necessary, then gently turn your partner's head to the right. Place your right hand on their forehead, or, if you prefer, support the head by letting it rest in your right hand. Place your left hand on your partner's left shoulder and glide your hand firmly all the way up to the neck.* ◀

2. *When you reach the base of the skull, use all your fingers and gently circle the area several times to release any muscle tension. Return to the gliding movement and repeat several times before slowly turning your partner's head to the left. Repeat the sequence on the right side.* ▶

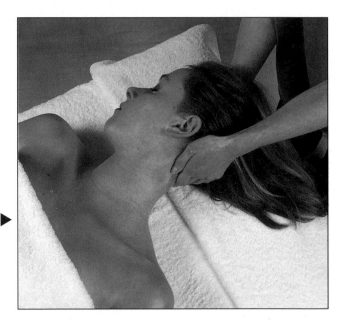

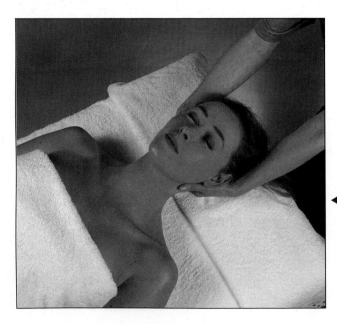

3. *Gently move your partner's head to the middle so that they are lying in a straight position once more. Now give the neck a good stretch. Clasp your hands together at the back of the neck and lift the head a few inches from the massage surface; pull from the base of the skull towards you. Still supporting your partner's head, allow it to come back* ◀ *down gently. Repeat several times.*

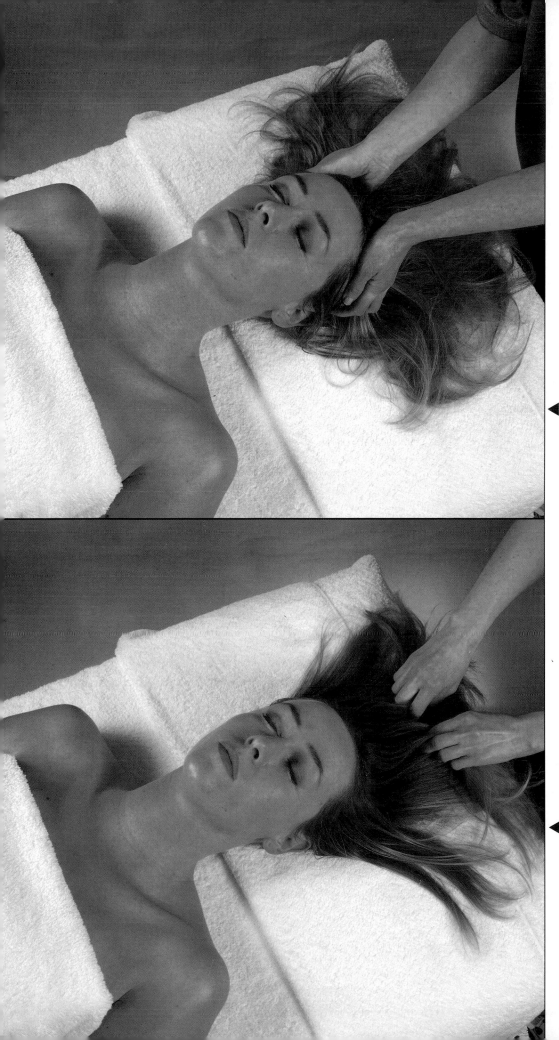

The Scalp

1. *Unless your partner is completely bald there is no need to oil the scalp. Using your fingers, press quite firmly and move your fingers and scalp over the bone. Do not simply slide your fingers through the hair over the scalp. Work up and down the head, covering the entire area.* ◀

2. *Run your fingers through your partner's hair several times, allowing your fingers to brush the scalp.*

Finish by holding your palms lightly against your partner's forehead with your fingers extending down the temples (see page 90). Hold your hands in this position for a few moments, then gently move away. ◀

Ending the Massage

Conclude with full-body feathering as described on page 59, but ensure that your partner is warmly covered with towels from neck to toe.

As an alternative, complete the entire massage sequence by holding: hold the feet for several seconds (place the palms of your hands over the soles of the feet), then the knees (place the palms of your hands over the kneecaps), then the hands (place the palms of your hands over the backs of your partner's hands) and finally the head and abdomen (place one hand on the forehead, the other lightly on the abdomen).

When you are ready, gently move away, allowing your partner to rest for a while and to 'come round' in their own time.

Massage for Elderly People

As we grow older, many of us suffer from coldness and stiffness in the joints and extremities, coupled with poor circulation. Regular massage and aromatic baths will improve skin and muscle tone, flexibility in the joints and the circulation, and may even prevent the onset of hypothermia.

It may be difficult to massage an elderly person on the floor, so if you do not have a massage table, sit the person astride a chair, facing its back. The recipient may, if they wish, lean forward against a cushion placed over the back of the chair. When you come to work on the lower back, kneel on the floor or sit in another chair of equal height.

Prepare a massage oil suitable for the person's needs (see the therapeutic charts in Chapter 7).

CAUTION
Caution: Do not massage anyone with advanced heart disease or inflammation of the joints (as in arthritis). Massage should only be carried out when the inflammation has calmed down, inflammation in joints tends to flare up and then die down continually.

Improving Flexibility and Circulation in the Hands and Feet

1. Stroke the foot and hand, then work in circles with your thumbs over the whole foot or hand, concentrating on the ankle or wrist joint. Work gently and intuitively, always massaging towards the heart to improve circulation.

2. Hold the ankle or wrist with one hand as you gently rotate the joint first clockwise, then anti-clockwise, with the other hand; but never cause pain. Regular massage will eventually allow free movement of the joint.

3. Repeat step one.

4. To ease stiffness in the finger and toe joints, gently stretch them to their point of resistance, again causing no pain, and rotate first clockwise then anti-clockwise.

When working on the feet, sit close to your partner and support the leg on a cushion placed on your lap, or allow the recipient to rest the foot on a padded stool of a similar height to their own chair.

The most comfortable way to work on the hands is to sit your partner in an armchair, resting their hands on the arms of the chair.

Additional Strokes

Tapotement (percussion)

Unlike other massage strokes, tapotement is stimulating rather than relaxing. It encompasses a range of brisk rhythmic strokes performed repeatedly with alternate hands. The main value of tapotement is to stimulate soft tissue areas such as thighs and buttocks, thus toning the skin and improving the circulation. It can also be helpful for breaking down cellulite, and is an excellent form of massage following strenuous exercise (but not if the muscles are painful). Although there are several other tapotement movements, we shall concentrate on the easiest to master – *pummelling*, *hacking* and *cupping*. Incidentally, before trying out the strokes on a partner, practise them on your own leg, ensuring that your hands are relaxed and your wrists loose. This can be achieved by giving your hands a good shake before you start.

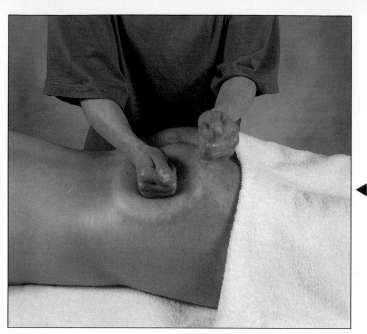

Pummelling
Loosely clench your fists, bouncing the fleshy sides of your fists alternately and rapidly against ◀ the skin.

Cupping
Cup your hands, arching them at the knuckles, fingers straight. Repeat the same rapid sequence of alternate strokes as before. Your cupped hands will trap air against the skin, then release it, making a sucking sound. Although hardly conducive to meditative massage, tapotement, ▶ especially cupping, usually makes people laugh! – a great tension-reliever.

After carrying out tapotement, always soothe the muscle by gently stroking the area with the whole of your hands.

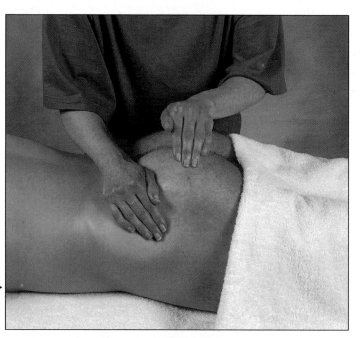

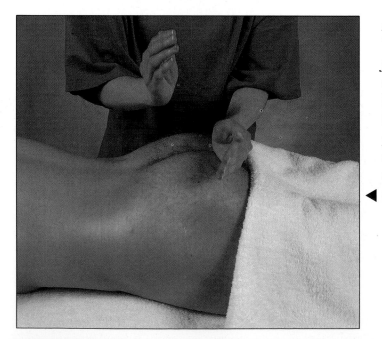

Hacking
With your palms facing each other, and your fingers loosely together, bounce the sides of your hands alternately and rapidly up ◀ and down.

Pressures

Deep pressure can help when there is pain, stiffness, or muscle spasm. It can be applied to the muscles either side of the spine and around the shoulders, and the buttock area. Use the ball of your thumb, your fingers, or the heel of your hand to apply the pressure in a circular motion, gradually and steadily leaning your weight into the movement. To reduce any discomfort your partner may feel as a result of finger pressure, try to synchronize your breathing, applying the pressure as you both breathe out, easing the pressure on the in-breath. Most important: even though the thumb, finger or the heel of the hand rotates as you apply the pressure, your hands should not move across the skin. The purpose of pressure is to cause the tissues beneath the skin to glide across the muscles, thus stimulating and warming the stiff or painful area.

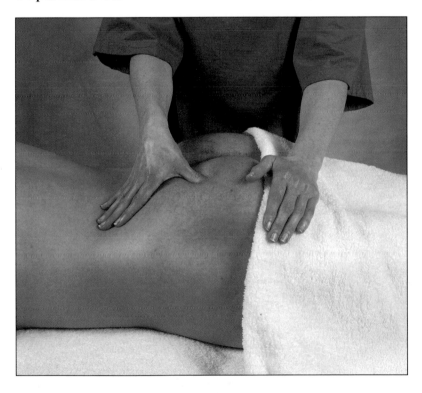

CAUTION – When Not to Apply Pressure
If pain is severe and/or seems to be related to a vital organ, seek medical advice as soon as possible.
Never use finger pressure massage on a mole, wart, varicose vein, swelling, inflammation, or a scar that has not completely healed.
Never apply pressure on the abdomen or on the breasts.
Never apply pressure during pregnancy.
Never apply pressure on fractured bones, torn ligaments, burns, cuts, or other trauma injuries.

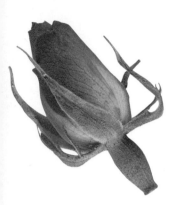

Self-Massage

When a willing friend is unavailable, you can derive much benefit from massaging aromatic oils into your own body. You will not be able to reach all areas, or be able to relax completely, but the advantages will outweigh the disadvantages. You can tailor the massage to suit your needs by using fast stimulating movements when you feel sluggish, and slow calming strokes when you feel tense.

Prepare an aromatherapy blend to suit your needs (see Chapter 4), then take a bath or shower. The oils penetrate the skin more readily when warm and slightly damp.

The direction of the movements should be towards the heart to encourage a good flow of blood, and therefore nutrients, to the area being treated. The only time it is beneficial to massage away from the heart is when you are in a very tense state. If so, then before you begin the main part of the massage, soothe and calm yourself by lightly brushing or 'feathering' (see page 59) with your fingertips, moving down the front of your body, and then down your arms and legs. You can repeat the feathering stroke later, employing it as a finalé to the main part of the massage.

Begin the massage on your legs. It is easier to do this whilst sitting. Stroke all the way up the leg from the foot to the upper thigh, lightly at first, gradually becoming firmer.

Once you have improved the circulation by firm stroking, you may begin gently and rhythmically to knead your hips, thighs and calves. Using each hand alternately, take hold of your flesh with the whole palm of your hand and fingers, pull away from the bones and squeeze as if you were kneading dough. Do not pinch or squeeze so hard that it causes pain – this will do no good and may result in bruising.

Stroke and knead your buttocks whilst standing or lying on your side. Try also to stroke oil over the whole of the lower and mid back. You will find this area easier to reach if you broad-circle the area using the back of your hand.

Sit down and work on your feet, referring to the foot massage sequence on pages 78–82, adapting the movements as necessary.

Stroke your whole arm from wrist to shoulder, then knead the forearm and the upper arm, gently squeezing and releasing the flesh. Using your thumb, apply circular pressures all over the forearm. Massage the area all around your elbow with your fingertips, using extra oil if necessary.

Now massage your hands, referring to the hand massage sequence on pages 86–88, adapting the movements as necessary.

Lie on your back with your knees bent and your feet flat on the floor, or stand up. Then massage your abdomen, using the whole of your hand and gently circle the area in a clockwise direction. This helps to prevent constipation by strengthening peristalsis (waves of contraction which move food through the intestines). Incidentally, essential oils are more easily absorbed into the bloodstream when massaged into this area and into the soft skin of the inner thighs and upper arms.

Sit or stand for the rest of the massage. Using the whole of your left hand, broadcircle the back of your neck and around the right shoulder blade. Then, starting at the base of your skull, stroke down the side of your neck, over your shoulder and down your arm to the elbow. Repeat several times. Then change hands, using the right hand to work on the opposite side of the neck and shoulder.

Now massage your face and ears, referring to the sequence described on pages 90–95, adapting the movements as necessary. You might also like to include the following additional strokes which are designed to further release tension around the eyes, to energize the lymphatic system and help keep nasal and sinus passages clear.

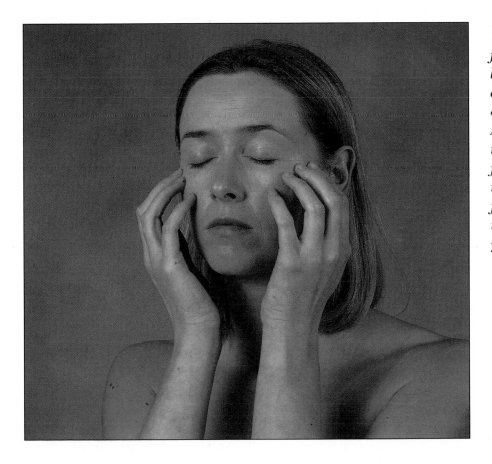

1. *Using your fingertips, drum lightly across your cheekbones and around your eyes. Allow your fingertips to reach across your forehead, then lightly tap all over the forehead, around the temples and into your hairline.*

2. *Close your eyes, and using your middle three fingertips, press lightly along the contours of the eye socket beneath the brow bone, working outwards. Then with your index fingers, lightly stroke the brow bone just beneath the eyebrow, working towards the temples. Repeat two or three times.* ▶

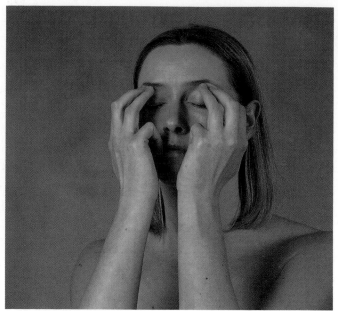

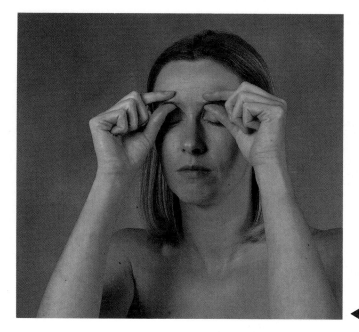

3. *With your index finger and thumb, squeeze all along the eyebrows, working from the nose out.* ◀ *Repeat several times.*

Now massage your scalp. If carried out two or three times a week for several months, scalp massage can help to stimulate hair growth by increasing the circulation and nourishment to the hair roots. There is no need to use any oil, unless you wish to use an aromatherapy pre-wash conditioning treatment (see the section on 'Aromatic Concoctions' in Chapter 7).

Shape your hands like a claw and push your fingers firmly into the scalp at the sides. Keeping your fingers in the same place so that you move the scalp over the bone rather than sliding your fingers across the surface, move in tiny circles. Continue all over your head until all parts of the scalp have been reached. Finish by 'shampooing' vigorously over your entire scalp. This time, rub your fingers across the surface of the scalp in order to loosen any flaky skin cells, then enjoy the pleasant tingling sensation!

Dry Skin Brushing

Skin brushing is a well-proven European 'nature cure' technique which could be described as a form of self lymphatic massage. (The lymphatic system is concerned with our immune defences – the production of antibodies against infection – and with the elimination of toxic wastes through the skin, lungs, kidneys and colon.) Skin brushing helps the condition of the skin itself by removing the build-up of dead skin cells on the surface, and it stimulates lymphatic drainage and the elimination of as much as one-third of body wastes. According to natural healing principles, these toxins can lead to disease if they are allowed to accumulate in the body. Complaints such as arthritis, cellulite, high blood pressure and even depression have all, at some time, been linked to poor lymphatic drainage.

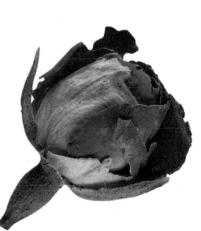

Skin brushing, then, is an all-round health treatment suitable for most people, especially if you lead a sedentary life, perhaps because you are wheel-chair bound, or you are elderly – or simply lazy! However, be careful if you suffer from a skin disorder such as eczema or psoriasis or if you have any infected or broken skin. Brush where the skin is healthy, and also avoid any areas where you have bad varicose veins.

Skin-brushing Technique

You will need a purpose-designed vegetable bristle brush (nylon or animal bristles are either too soft or too rough) with a long, but detachable handle so that you can reach your back. These are available from many health shops and a few chemists. The brush must be always kept dry but washed in warm soapy water every two weeks. Brush your body once a day for a few minutes before your morning bath or shower, twice daily if you have cellulite. Take a week's break every month as skin brushing, like many natural detoxification techniques, is more effective if the body does not become too accustomed to it.

Begin at the tips of your shoulders and cover your whole body with long sweeping strokes. Go downwards over the arms, shoulders and upper chest, avoiding the face and nipples, which are too sensitive for this treatment, and then upwards over the feet, legs and buttocks to the middle of the back. Always work towards the heart and bring toxins towards the colon. You will need to go over the skin only once or twice. Finally, brush the abdomen (avoiding the genitals), using a clockwise circular motion.

Maternity

You can enjoy gentle massage with plain vegetable oil throughout pregnancy, but do seek the approval of your doctor or midwife first.

Usually, during this time, unless you are under the guidance of a qualified aromatherapist, it is best to avoid essential oils in the bath and for massage. Essences can be vaporized (see page 44) instead. Choose from the following which are recommended for use during pregnancy:

bergamot, grapefruit, lavender, lemon, mandarin, neroli, orange, petitgrain, rose, pine, sandalwood, ylang-ylang.

If you are massaging a pregnant woman, it is important to avoid deep pressures and percussion strokes such as pummelling and hacking. In the later stages of pregnancy, when she is unable to lie on her front, you can massage her back whilst she lies on her side or sits astride a chair. Pay special attention to her legs, especially the thighs, which can become quite tense during pregnancy. You can gently and smoothly massage her abdomen by stroking the whole area in broad clockwise circles, gradually becoming lighter and lighter until you are barely touching the skin. This has a soporific effect on mother and baby. Overall, massage during pregnancy helps reduce fluid retention and aids deeper sleep. Mothers-to-be have also noticed that they develop fewer, if any stretchmarks by massaging with extra virgin olive oil.

During Childbirth

Essential oils can be an enormous help during labour. Indeed, a growing number of maternity units, including the John Radcliffe maternity unit in Oxford, are now offering aromatherapy to soothe both mother and baby during the birthing process.

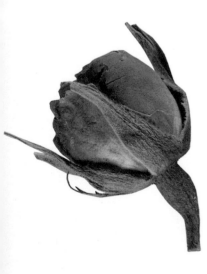

A blend of lavender, chamomile and clary sage massaged into the lower back reduces pain and speeds up labour. During the transition phase – the shortest yet most painful stage of labour – the same blend can be gently massaged into the abdomen using circular strokes. Apply minimal pressure, as it is the lightness of touch that soothes the underlying muscles.

A drop or two of frankincense and rose, inhaled as required from the palm of the hand, has been successfully used at the John Radcliffe unit to help women suffering from hyperventilation (over breathing) during labour. In addition, clary sage helps with the delivery of the placenta (afterbirth) when used as a warm compress over the abdomen.

Some women experience shaking legs at the end of the first stage of labour, and also immediately after giving birth. This can be helped by stroking the thighs from the upper part to the knee and back again. Press firmly down the leg, and lightly as you move upwards. Always keep your movements flowing and rhythmic.

Nursing Mothers

Because essential oils are easily absorbed into the bloodstream and body fluids and so can end up in the mother's milk, you are advised to continue to play safe when breastfeeding. Whilst there is no documented evidence to suggest that babies have been harmed, it is best to err on the side of caution, and, throughout pregnancy and breastfeeding, not to over-use any perfumed product, especially skin perfumes. The latter contain a high concentration of volatile aroma chemicals which, like essential oils, easily penetrate the skin and find their way into the bloodstream and other bodily fluids.

A weekly massage, however, with half-to-one per cent concentrations of carefully chosen essential oils (see opposite for those recommended especially for pregnancy) is perfectly safe and beneficial for both mother and baby. Alternatively, use a plain base oil for massage and vaporize your favourite essential oils.

Incidentally, many nursing mothers have reported to me that geranium essence has a stimulating effect on the baby, so it may be advisable to avoid this oil if you wish to get a good night's sleep! Also, it is best to avoid peppermint in any shape or form whilst breastfeeding – herbalists have always used this to help decrease the flow of milk. However, fennel and lemongrass (both the herb and the essential oil) stimulate the flow.

Babies

In recent years, natural childbirth gurus such as Frederick Leboyer of *Birth Without Violence* fame, and Michel Odent of birthing-in-water fame, have revived the ancient art of baby massage. In parts of the East and in many tropical countries, baby massage is regarded as one of the essential skills of motherhood, and is passed down from mother to daughter. Massage is believed to help babies grow stronger by encouraging deep sleep, better feeding and the relief of colic. Many Western psychologists and paediatricians also believe it encourages bonding and communication between mother and baby, and many enlightened fathers massage their babies, too.

In babies and young children, the sense of smell is especially acute, and, although some aromatherapists advocate the use of essential oils diluted in almond oil for baby massage, I feel it is safer to use only plain almond oil, particularly if your baby is under twelve months. After this age, you may safely add **one drop** of chamomile or lavender to 25ml of almond oil. Alternatively, by vaporizing a low concentration of essential oils such as lavender, neroli, rose, bergamot and other citrus essences, you could perfume the room in which you intend to give the massage.

Massaging your Baby

From the first week after the birth, you can start rubbing your baby lightly with oil. Try to massage your baby every day, perhaps just before bathtime. As the baby grows a little older, he or she will take an active part in the massage, wriggling, kicking and gurgling in response to your touch. So make it a game between the two of you!

When massaging, Indian mothers sit on the floor with their legs outstretched to form a cradle in which they lay their babies. If you find this position uncomfortable, support your back with cushions propped against the wall. Alternatively, massage your baby on your lap whilst sitting in bed, or whilst kneeling on a carpeted floor with your baby on a towel. Remember to cover your lap (or the floor) and the surrounding area with a few extra towels – just in case! Ensure that the room is very warm.

Begin on the front of the body. Slowly and gently rub a little oil all over the baby's body, shoulders to feet, but avoid the face to prevent the possibility of oil seeping into the eyes.

1. *Starting from baby's hips, slide your hands up to the shoulders, then down the sides of the body. Repeat several times.*

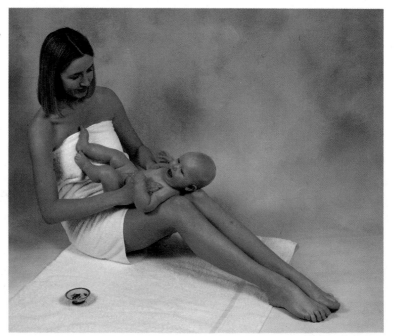

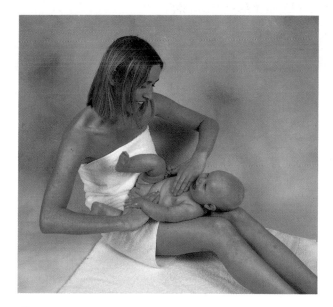

2. *Next massage baby's tummy, stroking clockwise around the navel with one hand following the other. Lift one hand over your other arm as your arms cross. Repeat several times.* ▲

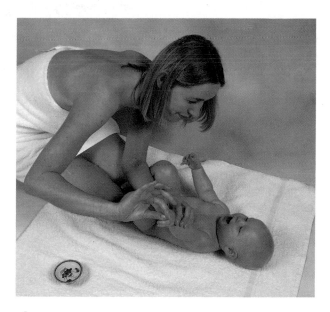

4. *Stroke the back of baby's hand, and then the palm. Gently squeeze and rotate each finger. Repeat the sequence on the other arm and hand.* ▲

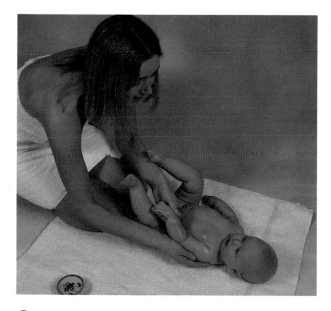

3. *Hold baby's hand in one hand, and stroke down the arm from shoulder to wrist, then gently squeeze all the way down the arm. Repeat several times.* ▲

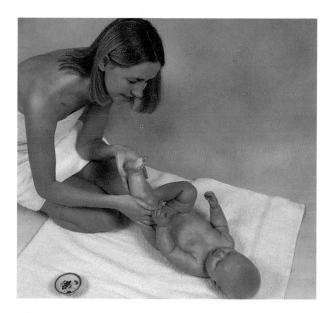

5. *Holding baby's foot in one hand, stroke the leg from thigh to ankle, then gently squeeze the leg all the way down. Repeat several times. Stroke the foot, front and sole, then squeeze and rotate each toe. Then work on the other leg and foot.* ▲

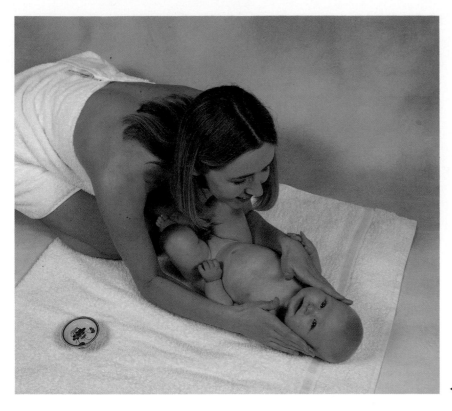

6. *If your baby is happy with face massage, then massage the face. There is no need to use more oil – that which is left on your hands from the body massage will be enough.*

Stroke baby's forehead with your thumbs, starting from the centre and smoothing outwards. Then stroke from either side of the nose to the temples. Using your middle fingers, very gently and lightly circle around baby's eyes, stroking out along the eyebrows, pressing softly on the temples. Place your thumbs above the upper lip and circle them around the ◀ *mouth in opposite directions, meeting on the chin. Repeat two or three times.*

7. *Turn the baby over and oil the back of the body. Stroke up the back of the legs, over the buttocks and up the back. Slide your hands across the shoulders and down the arms, then pull them gently down the sides.* ▶

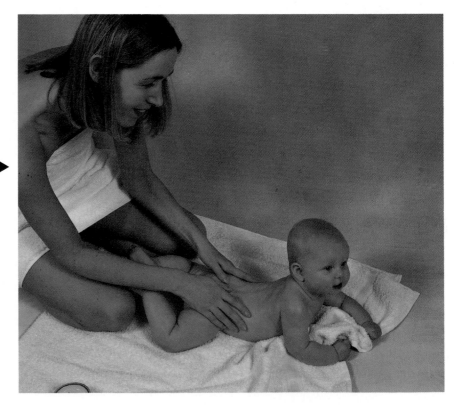

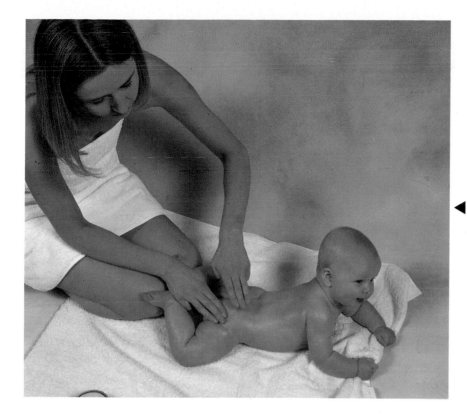

8. *Stroke each buttock, then very gently knead, using either your thumbs and fingers, or two hands to gently press the entire buttocks together.*

Babies also love their bottom patted, so with four fingers of one hand, gently pat all over the buttocks. ◀

9. *Finish the massage by sliding your hands very gently and smoothly down the back, one hand following the other. As one hand reaches the legs, lift it off, return to the top of the back and repeat. Gradually stroke more and more slowly and lightly. This smooth continuous stroke has a calming, soporific effect.* ▶

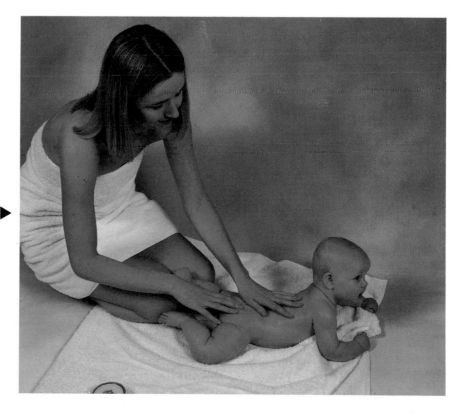

As a baby's body is so small, you will tend to use the stroking movements most often. The following simple massage sequence does not have to be done 'by the book', just do whatever your baby enjoys. Some babies dislike face massage, for instance, although most appreciate having their forehead stroked.

Massaging Children

Children enjoy aromatherapy massage as much as adults. For children between the ages of five-to-ten years, use the lowest concentration of essential oil, between half-to-one per cent for massage and no more than three drops in the bath water. Alternatively, vaporize their favourite oils. Children tend to choose floral or citrus essences, especially lavender, rose, mandarin, and bergamot.

CAUTION
Most massage strokes, except deep pressure, can be used on children.
Avoid percussion strokes on children under five years old.
Avoid using essential oils on the face if your child is under ten years old, and use, instead, a little plain almond or extra virgin olive oil, keeping well away from the eye area.

Although children love being massaged, they may not lie still for more than ten minutes, twenty minutes at the most. From my own experience, they wriggle and giggle at first, but after a while even a hyperactive child settles down. Set out to do a shortened version of the full-body massage described in Chapter 5, gently stroking and kneading according to your child's preference. Alternatively, concentrate on a back and/or foot massage. If carried out after your child's evening bath, even ten minutes' quality massage will ensure a good night's sleep.

As you will discover, massaging babies and children is fun for both giver and recipient, so relax and enjoy it!

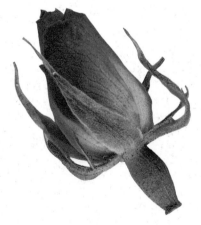

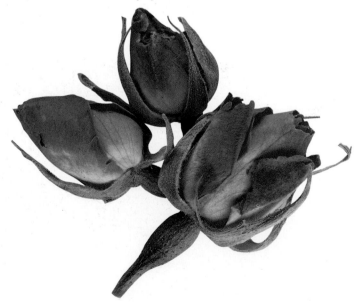

Therapeutic and Aesthetic Blending

Over the next few pages you will find therapeutic cross reference charts that suggests essential oils and their methods of application for a number of common ailments. The list, however, is in no way comprehensive. Aromatherapy – complemented by a healthy diet and lifestyle – can prevent and alleviate a great many more health problems than are mentioned in this chapter.

Other supportive measures, such as herbal remedies (see 'Preparing Herbal Medicines', page 118) and nutritional supplements are also recommended where appropriate. The charts are best used as an at-a-glance-reference, supported by the essential oil profiles in Chapter 3, and the methods and techniques of aromatherapy as described in subsequent chapters.

The final part of this chapter offers a number of aromatherapeutic recipes just to get you started on the fragrant path.

Herbal Medicines

Instead of taking essences by mouth to help certain health problems (as advocated by some aromatherapists), I have suggested herbal remedies where appropriate. It is best for the lay person to avoid internal doses of essential oils because they are potentially harmful if unwisely administered. The herbal remedies suggested in the charts on pages 114–117 are safe to use if you follow the correct procedure for preparation and administer the recommended dosage. Loose medicinal herbs are available from herbalists and many health shops. Alternatively, instead of preparing your own medicinal brews, herbal medicines are available in tablet form from the same outlets.

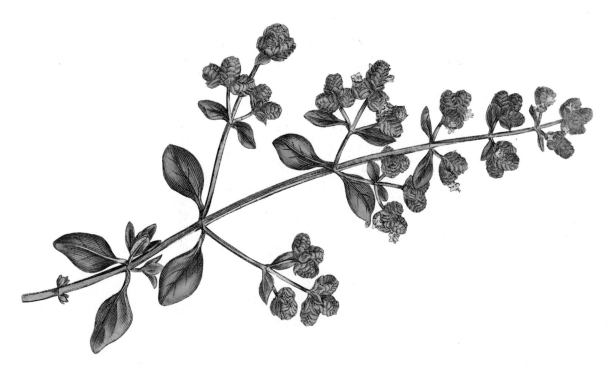

ESSENTIAL OILS

PROBLEM	Basil	Bergamot	Black Pepper	Cedarwood	Chamomile, Roman	Clary Sage	Coriander	Cypress	Eucalyptus	Frankincense	Geranium	Ginger	Grapefruit	Juniper	Lavender	Lemon	Marjoram, Sweet	Myrrh	Neroli or Orange Blossom	Orange
CIRCULATION — Cellulite				✿				✿			✿		✿	✿	✿	✿				
Circulation, poor			✿				✿	✿				✿		✿	✿	✿	✿			✿
Chilblains			✿		✿						✿				✿	✿				
DIGESTION — Constipation			✿														✿			
FIRST AID — Bruises															✿		✿			
Burns & scalds											✿				✿					
Sprains					✿				✿			✿			✿		✿			
Insect bites & stings									✿						✿					
Wounds, cuts & grazes					✿				✿	✿	✿				✿	✿				
HEAD — Dandruff					✿	✿			✿					✿	✿					
Head lice									✿		✿				✿					
MENSTRUAL — Menopause (hot flushes, mood swings)		✿			✿	✿		✿			✿				✿				✿	✿
Menstrual cramps					✿	✿		✿				✿		✿	✿		✿			
Menstruation, delayed	✿				✿	✿								✿			✿	✿		
Menstruation, excessive								✿			✿									
PMS (pre-menstrual syndrome)		✿			✿	✿	✿	✿			✿			✿	✿	✿			✿	✿

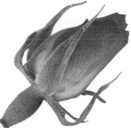

Patchouli	Peppermint	Petitgrain	Pine, Scots	Rose Otto	Rosemary	Sandalwood	Tea Tree	Vetiver	Ylang-Ylang	METHOD	FURTHER SUGGESTIONS
✿					✿					Baths, massage.	A diet high in raw fruit and vegetables; plenty of fresh air and exercise. Dry skin brushing (see p105). Herbal remedies: vervain, nettle.
				✿	✿				✿	Baths, massage.	If physically able, adequate exercise, deep breathing. Herbal remedies: thyme, yarrow.
										Baths, hand/footbaths, essential oil ointment.	For ointment recipe, see p122, 'Aromatic Concoctions'. For broken chilblains: apply neat lavender. (See also advice for 'Poor Circulation' above).
				✿	✿					Baths, massage (especially over abdomen using circular strokes, clockwise direction following colon).	Ensure that your diet is high in fruits, vegetables and wholegrains. Drink plenty of warm spring water on rising. Take adequate exercise in the fresh air and seek to reduce stress.
										Cold compress, essential oil ointment.	For ointment recipe see p122 'Aromatic Concoctions'.
										Apply neat to small burns, as a cold compress to larger burns.	Cool burns and scalds immediately under cold, running water. Serious burns and scalds need urgent medical attention.
	✿				✿		✿			Cold compress, essential oil ointment.	See ointment recipe, p122 'Aromatic Concoctions'.
							✿			Apply neat or incorporated into an ointment.	See ointment recipe p122 'Aromatic Concoctions'.
✿							✿	✿		Apply neat lavender eucalyptus or tea tree, or add 10 drops to 50ml of water and sprinkle on a lint dressing.	To aid healing, apply an essential oil ointment; see recipe p122 'Aromatic Concoctions'.
				✿			✿			Scalp massage, hair and scalp oil, hair tonic.	If severe, appearing thick and greasy, seek dietry advice from a nutritionist or holistic therapist (see also 'Aromatic Concoctions' p119).
				✿			✿			Hair oil.	See p119 'Aromatic Concoctions'.
		✿		✿		✿		✿	✿	Use cypress, clary sage, geranium & chamomile in baths or massage, use others in skin or room perfumes.	Deep breathing, yoga, fresh air and excercise, Herbal remedies: black cohosh, chaste tree, sage (for hot flushes and night sweats) Seek professional help if symptoms are severe.
				✿						Massage over back & abdomen throughout cycle. Warm compress during menstruation. Use oils in bath.	Herbal remedies: black cohosh, chaste tree, marigold.
				✿						Baths, massage, warm compress.	Ensure that you are not excessively over or underweight. Seek to reduce stress. Herbal remedies: chaste tree, pennyroyal, marigold.
				✿						Regular massage, particularly to the lower back. Baths.	Seek medical advice if symptoms persist. Herbal remedies: cranesbill, lady's mantle.
✿		✿		✿		✿		✿	✿	Baths, massage, skin and room perfumes.	Efamol (evening primrose oil with zinc, B6, magnesium and vitamin C). Available as a pre-menstrual pack from chemists and health shops. Seek to reduce stress. Herbal remedy: chaste tree.

ESSENTIAL OILS

PROBLEM		Basil	Bergamot	Black Pepper	Cedarwood	Chamomile, Roman	Clary Sage	Coriander	Cypress	Eucalyptus	Frankincense	Geranium	Ginger	Grapefruit	Juniper	Lavender	Lemon	Marjoram, Sweet	Myrrh	Neroli or Orange Blossom	Orange
MOUTH	Gingivitis								❀										❀		
MOUTH	Mouth ulcers								❀			❀							❀		
MUSCLE & JOINTS	Arthritis & rheumatism					❀		❀	❀	❀			❀		❀	❀	❀	❀			
MUSCLE & JOINTS	Muscles, over-worked, aching		❀	❀		❀		❀	❀	❀			❀		❀	❀		❀			
RESPIRATORY	Colds, 'flu, sinusitis, coughs	❀		❀	❀				❀	❀			❀	❀	❀	❀	❀	❀	❀		❀
RESPIRATORY	Catarrh				❀	❀				❀	❀		❀			❀			❀		
SKIN	Acne		❀		❀	❀			❀	❀		❀			❀	❀				❀	
SKIN	Athlete's foot															❀			❀		
SKIN	Eczema				❀	❀						❀				❀					
SKIN	Scabies															❀					
SKIN	Ringworm											❀									
STRESS-RELATED	Anxiety	❀	❀		❀	❀	❀		❀		❀	❀			❀	❀		❀	❀	❀	❀
STRESS-RELATED	Depression	❀	❀			❀	❀	❀			❀	❀		❀	❀	❀				❀	❀
STRESS-RELATED	Insomnia					❀	❀		❀		❀	❀			❀	❀		❀		❀	
STRESS-RELATED	Headache	❀				❀										❀		❀			

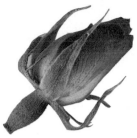

Patchouli	Peppermint	Petitgrain	Pine, Scots	Rose Otto	Rosemary	Sandalwood	Tea Tree	Vetiver	Ylang-Ylang	METHOD	FURTHER SUGGESTIONS
							✿			Mouthwash.	Visit your dentist! (See mouthwash recipe, p121, 'Aromatic Concoctions').
							✿			Mouthwash, see recipe p121.	Seek to reduce stress; take 1g of vitamin C daily and a strong B-complex formula.
			✿		✿					Baths, massage, foot/hand baths where appropriate (alternate **hot & cold**, finish with **cold.**)	Diet is very important. It's advisable to seek the advice of a nutritionist &/or holistic therapist. Never massage *inflamed* joints – it's too painful to do so anyway. Fresh air, sunshine, swimming in the sea & spa baths help. Herbal remedies: devil's claw.
✿			✿		✿					Baths, massage, warm compress.	
✿			✿			✿	✿			Baths, foot/bath, inhalations, massage oil as a chest rub. Room perfume/fumigant: clove & cinnamon.	**1.** For colds & 'flu: honey, lemon & grated ginger root(to taste) in hot water, 3 x daily. **2.** As a preventative remedy for respiratory ailments, take 2 garlic capsules & 2 x 500mg vitamin C daily. **3.** Coughs/sore throats: 2 drops lavender, cypress or eucalyptus in a teacup of warm water to be used as a gargle 3 x daily.
✿		✿	✿	✿	✿					Baths, inhalation, massage.	For chronic catarrh, seek the advice of a holistic therapist. Try to cut down on dairy products. Herbal remedies: yarrow, lemon balm, peppermint.
✿				✿	✿	✿	✿		✿	Facial oils &/or skin tonics, facial sauna, body massage, baths.	Holistic treatment is essential. Seek the advice of a qualified aromatherapist. Herbal remedies: dandelion, burdock, horsetail, nettle.
✿							✿			Apply neat to affected parts or use essential oil ointment. Footbaths. Sprinkle oils on hosiery & in shoes.	Expose feet to fresh air and sunshine as often as possible. Keep feet dry and scrupulously clean. For ointment recipe, see p122 'Aromatic Concoctions'.
					✿					Baths, general massage (not over the affected areas), essential oil ointment.	For chronic cases, holistic treatment is essential. Seek advice. Herbal remedies: chamomile red clover, nettle, marigold. (See 'Aromatic Concoctions' for ointment recipe, p122.)
	✿			✿			✿			Essential oil ointment, baths.	Apply ointment 3 x daily & take 3-6 garlic capsules daily until cleared. Scabies is contagious, boil towels/linen & do not share with others (see ointment recipe, p122 'Aromatic Concoctions'.)
	✿						✿			Essential oil ointment.	Apply ointment 3 x daily. (See recipe, p122 'Aromatic Concoctions'.)
✿		✿		✿	✿			✿	✿	Baths, massage, skin and room perfume.	Long-term anxiety needs the help of a professional counsellor or holistic therapist. Herbal remedies: Bach Flower Remedies (available from many health shops).
✿		✿		✿	✿				✿	Baths, massage, skin and room perfume.	As for anxiety.
		✿		✿	✿			✿	✿	Baths, massage, skin and room perfume.	As for anxiety & depression, plus the following herbal remedies: valerian, hops, passion flower, wild lettuce.
	✿			✿	✿					Head, face & neck massage. Sniff a few drops of peppermint. Migraine headaches: use cold compress.	The many causes of headache are too numerous to mention here. For continual migraine-type headaches seek medical advice. Herbal remedies: peppermint, chamomile, skullcap, rosemary.

Preparing Herbal Medicines

✳ Infusion (tea)

Put 15g dried herbs into a warmed china or pyrex vessel. Pour over 600ml of boiling water and allow to steep for ten-to-fifteen minutes. If using fresh herbs, you will generally need three times as much. Seeds such as fennel should be bruised to release the essential oils from the cells before being made into an infusion.

Dosage

The usual dosage is a wine glass three times a day every four hours.

✳ Decoction

*This is used for hard woody plant material such as roots, rhizomes and barks. Put 15g of dried plant material, or 45g of fresh, broken into small pieces, into an enamel saucepan or other heatproof vessel. **Never use aluminium** as poisonous seepage will react with the plant alkaloids and its vitamin content, thus damaging the therapeutic properties. Pour over 300ml of water and simmer with the lid on for ten-to-fifteen minutes.*

Dosage

Same as an infusion.

Aromatic Concoctions

The following recipes are a selection of my own aromatic concoctions; no doubt you will invent many more!

Baths and Massage Oils

The following blends of essential oils are suitable for therapeutic baths as indicated. To make a corresponding massage oil, simply double the quantity of essential oil and mix with 20ml-to-30ml of a base oil of your choice. If you wish to adapt the blends to suit your own preference, try not to greatly exceed the total number of drops suggested.

✳ To Aid Restful Sleep

Blend 1 – *lavender 2, juniper 1, sandalwood 3.*

Blend 2 – *chamomile 1, neroli 2, clary sage 3.*

Blend 3 – *rose otto 1, petitgrain 3.*

✳ For Muscular Aches and Pains, Colds and 'Flu

Blend 1 – **(stimulating)** *rosemary 3, bergamot 3, ginger 2.*

Blend 2 – **(relaxing)** *lavender 2, marjoram 2, bergamot 2, chamomile 1.*

Blend 3 – **(medicinal aroma)** *eucalyptus 2, tea tree 3, pine 2.*

❋ For Treating Cellulite

Blend 1 – *lemon 3, cypress 3, patchouli 1.*
Blend 2 – *juniper 3, lavender 1, rosemary 3.*
Blend 3 – *orange 3, pine 4.*

❋ Three Special Blends

Blend 1 – *bergamot 3, clary sage 2, ylang-ylang 2.*
Use when you feel tense with worrying thoughts constantly invading your sleep.
Blend 2 – *sandalwood 3, bergamot 2, grapefruit 2.*
Use when you need comforting and uplifting.
Blend 3 – *patchouli (or vetiver) 2, ginger 1, orange (or coriander) 4.*
Use when you feel ungrounded, especially after a bout of 'flu when you may be feeling light-headed and distant.

❋ Treatment for Head Lice

75ml any vegetable oil
25 drops tea tree or eucalyptus
25 drops lavender
25 drops rosemary

Funnel the vegetable oil into a dark glass bottle, add the essential oils and shake well.

How to use
Apply to wet hair (otherwise it will be difficult to shampoo out the oil) by massaging well into the scalp to reach the hair roots. Pay particular attention to the areas around the ears and nape of the neck where the lice breed. Leave on for about an hour, then shampoo thoroughly. Remove the eggs (nits) with a regulation fine-toothed comb. Repeat twice at three-day intervals.

❋ Oil Treatment for Dandruff

50ml extra virgin olive oil
10 drops rosemary
10 drops lavender
5 drops tea tree or juniper

Mix as for previous recipe.

How to use
Apply to wet hair; massage into the scalp; and leave on for fifteen-to-thirty minutes. Shampoo thoroughly. Use as a weekly treatment. If your hair is oily, use an anti-dandruff hair tonic instead.

Hair Tonics

These are massaged into the scalp several times a week. There is no need to wet your hair first. If used regularly, they will improve the condition of your hair and scalp. Cider vinegar is included in all the recipes to restore the acid/alkali balance of the scalp. All hair tonics need to be shaken before use to disperse the essences.

✳ Anti-dandruff Tonic

300ml distilled water or 50/50 distilled water and witch hazel
3 teaspoons cider vinegar
6 drops lavender
6 drops rosemary
3 drops juniper or tea tree

Funnel the distilled water and cider vinegar into a dark glass, add the essences and shake well.

✳ Tonic for Thinning Hair

While this tonic may not be a cure for male-pattern baldness, if used regularly with scalp massage, it may halt the process.

300ml rosewater or distilled water
3 teaspoons cider vinegar
7 drops rosemary
5 drops sandalwood

Mix as for previous recipe.

✳ Skin Tonic Base

As for hair tonics, you will need to shake this well before use to disperse the essential oils. Apply once or twice a day after cleansing to tone the complexion.

You will need 300ml of rosewater (for normal, combination or oily skin) or orange flower water (normal-to-dry skin) or distilled water (all skin types).

For very oily skin or acne, you could use a more astringent base such as witch hazel. This could be made slightly less astringent by mixing it 50/50 with a flower water or distilled water.

To the flower water or distilled water base, add 2 teaspoons of cider vinegar, then add 2 or 3 drops of the appropriate essential oil for your skin type (refer to the Skin Care Chart in Chapter 4, page 42).

✳ **Mouthwash**

This is a healing, antiseptic mixture to strengthen the gums. It will also help to heal mouth ulcers and prevent the onset of gingivitis.

Base – *30ml tincture of myrrh (available from herbalists),* 10 drops peppermint or cypress or tea tree.

How to use – 6-to-8 drops in a small teacupful of warm water two or three times a day.

Making Skin Creams and Ointments

The following recipe makes a fairly soft cream which will harden slightly if kept in the fridge (to halt the formation of mould), but nevertheless melts on contact with the skin. As it is so rich, a tiny amount will go a long way, so do not be tempted to make a larger quantity than suggested here, unless you intend to share it with your friends. Use it as a hand-cream or face-cream for drier skin. It should keep for three-to-four months.

✳ **Skin Cream**

15g yellow beeswax
120ml almond oil (or the same quantity of any other fine vegetable oil)
30ml distilled water or rosewater or orange flower water
4-to-6 drops of essential oil (see skin care chart, page 42).

Melt the beeswax with the oil in a heatproof basin over a pan of simmering water.

Meanwhile, heat the distilled water in another basin over a pan of simmering water until it has warmed.

Begin to add the warm distilled water, drop by drop at first, to the oil and wax, beating with a rotary whisk or an electric food mixer set at medium to low speed.

After you have mixed about two teaspoons of the water into the oil and wax, remove from the heat and continue adding the water a little at a time until you have incorporated it all. As soon as the mixture begins to set, stir in the essences. (This is important because if the essential oil is added whilst the mixture is still very warm, it will quickly evaporate.)

Divide the mixture into little sterilized pots and cover tightly.

✳ Healing Ointment

15g yellow beeswax
60ml almond oil
20 drops of appropriate essential oil (see pages 114–117)

Heat the beeswax and almond oil in a heatproof dish over a pan of simmering water. Stir well, remove from the heat and cool, add the essential oils. Pour into a sterilized glass pot and cover tightly.

Important
For infectious skin problems, such as athlete's foot, scabies and ringworm, you will need to double the quantity of essential oil. A blend of lavender, tea tree and eucalyptus is a good choice for most problems. This ointment will keep for six-to-nine months (possibly longer) due to the high concentration of essential oils.

✳ Alternative healing recipe

You could 'doctor' an unperfumed shop-bought skin cream or ointment with the appropriate essential oils. To make an all-purpose antiseptic cream, add 20 drops in all to 30g of cream, stir in with the handle of a teaspoon.

Fun Blends

Aromatic Waters and Perfumes

Here you can become wild and creative, concocting exotic, relaxing or simple herbal blends as your moods dictate.

The aromatic waters can be used in the same way as shop-bought products – splashed on after a bath or shower. Natural perfumes need to be diluted in jojoba oil which is actually a liquid wax. Jojoba has a long shelf-life and is virtually odourless. Commercial perfumes and aromatic waters are diluted in ethyl alcohol which is not generally available without a perfumer's licence. Jojoba is not only kind to the skin, it also holds the fragrance of essential oils for much longer than alcohol or water.

✳ How to Make an Aromatic Water

Basic Procedure
100ml rosewater or orange flower water or distilled water
100 drops essential oil

Funnel the water base into a dark glass bottle, add the essential oils and shake well. Leave to stand for a week in a cool dark place to mature, then filter through a coffee filter paper before re-bottling.

Suggested Formulae

Mandelay – (an oriental-type aroma, very cheering and seductive).
To the flower water or distilled water base, add 16 drops ylang-ylang, 40 drops bergamot, 30 drops patchouli, 9 drops coriander, 1 drop ginger.

✻ Eau De Cologne

Classic
40 drops bergamot, 10 drops petitgrain, 10 drops orange, 25 drops lemon, 10 drops lavender, 5 drops rosemary.

Luxury
15 drops neroli, 4 drops rose otto, 15 drops grapefruit, 10 drops lemon, 30 drops bergamot, 14 drops mandarin, 10 drops orange.

Spicy
20 drops bergamot, 20 drops orange, 10 drops lavender, 10 drops coriander, 10 drops frankincense, 10 drops petitgrain, 5 drops lime.

✻ Perfumes

Using a 10ml base of jojoba, follow the basic procedure for perfume-making on page 50. Experiment with your own blends or try one of the concoctions overleaf.

Massage Oils

Dilute with 25ml of base oil

Starburst

Mandarin 2 drops
Geranium 2 drops
Black pepper 3 drops
Ylang-ylang 3 drops

Wood Nymph

Neroli 3 drops
Clary sage 2 drops
Juniper 2 drops
Cedarwood 3 drops

Adonis

Lemon 4 drops
Rose otto 2 drops
Sandalwood 4 drops

Joie de Vivre

Lavender 3 drops
Bergamot 3 drops
Coriander 2 drops
Neroli 2 drops

Perfumes

Dilute with 10ml of jojoba oil

I Return

Bergamot 6 drops
Orange 2 drops
Petitgrain 2 drops
Frankincense 5 drops

Truly, Madly, Deeply

Geranium 3 drops
Black pepper 4 drops
Rose otto 2 drops
Ylang-ylang 6 drops

Eternally Yours

Lavender 4 drops
Rose otto 2 drops
Patchouli 5 drops
Sandalwood 5 drops

Earth Spirit

Lavender 4 drops
Clary sage 5 drops
Petitgrain 3 drops
Vetiver 3 drops

Room Perfumes

Dilute in 30ml of water

Spring Maiden

Bergamot 5 drops
Rose otto 1 drop
Geranium 2 drops
Ylang-ylang 2 drops

Ode to Summer

Grapefruit 3 drops
Mandarin 3 drops
Black pepper 2 drops
Ylang-ylang 2 drops

Autumn Fruits

Mandarin 3 drops
Coriander 3 drops
Bergamot 2 drops
Vetiver 2 drops

Winter Spice

Lavender 3 drops
Coriander 6 drops
Ginger 1 drop
Clove 1 drop
Frankincense 2 drops

Aromatic Baths

Add to bath water

Sea of Tranquillity

Clary sage 3 drops
Vetiver 3 drops

Making Waves

Lemon 1 drop
Rosemary 4 drops
Peppermint 1 drop

Sweet Dreams

Chamomile 2 drops
Clary sage 2 drops
Neroli 2 drops

Siren

Coriander 3 drops
Rose otto 1 drop
Sandalwood 2 drops

A Final Wish

May you enjoy many timeless moments of giving and receiving nurturing massage, enhanced by the soul-caressing properties of plant essences — a precious gift from the fragrant Earth.

Further Reading

Arcier, M. *Aromatherapy*, Book Club Associates, 1990
Dougans, I. with Ellis, S. *Reflexology*, Element Books, 1991
Downing, G. *The Massage Book*, Penguin Books, 1982
Earl, L. *Save Your Skin with Vital Oils*, Vermilion, 1992
Maury, M. *The Secret of Life and Youth*, C.W. Daniel, 1989
Maxwell-Hudson, C. *The Complete Book of Massage*, Dorling Kindersley, 1990
Tisserand, R. *The Art of Aromatherapy*, C.W. Daniel, 1983
Wildwood, C. *Creative Aromatherapy*, Thorsons, 1993

Useful Addresses

Essential Oil Suppliers

The following suppliers stock a range of high quality aromatherapy grade oils and vaporizing equipment:

Kittywake Oils
Cae Kitty
Taliaris
Llandeilo
Dyfed SA9 7DP

Butterbur & Sage
101 Highgrove Street
Reading
Berks RG 5EJ

Aromatherapy Courses and Oils

Purple Flame Aromatics
61 Clinton Lane
Kenilworth
Warwickshire CV8 1AS

Aromatherapy Courses

The London School of Aromatherapy
PO Box 780
London NW5 1DY

Massage Courses

Clare Maxwell-Hudson
87 Dartmouth Road
London NW2 4BR

United States of America
Aroma Vera Inc.
PO Box 3609
Culver City
California 90231

Neal's Yard USA
284 Connecticut St
San Francisco
California 94107

United States of America
American AromaTherapy
Association
PO Box 1222, Fair Oaks
California 95628

Australia
Berida Manor
PO Box 350
Bowral
New South Wales 2576

For a list of accredited aromatherapists in your area, contact:

The International Federation of Aromatherapists
Department of Consulting Education
Royal Masonic Hospital
London W6 0TN

Please enclose a stamped addressed envelope with all enquiries.

Index

neck, 58, *66-7*, **90-6**
oils (*see* oils)
for pregnant women,
106
push-and-pull stroke,
76
scalp, *97*
self, **102-5**, *103*, *104*,
105
shoulderblade, *68*
shoulders, 58, *66*, *67*,
90-5
surface, **53-4**
Swedish, 55
techniques, 13-14, **55-105**
additional strokes, 99
ankle, *73*
back, *61*, 65
back glide, *61*
buttocks, *61*, *73*
circular movements,
65
cupping, 99, *100*
feathering, *59*
friction, *64*
gliding stroke, *60-1*,
65
hacking, 54, 99, *100*,
106
kneading, 55, *62*, *66-7*
neck, *66*, *67*
percussion *see*
Tapotement
pressures, *101*
pulling, *63*
pummelling, 54, 99,
100, 106
push-and-pull, *76*
riding the waves, *69*
shoulders, *66*, *67*
tapotement, 54-5, 99,
106, 112
thighs, *72*
timing the, **56**
when not to give a, **54**
maternity, babies and
children, **106-12**
Maury, Marguerite, **13**
measures, easy oil, **39**
medicinal essences, 37
medicine, western, 10
meditation, 45
Melaleuca alternifolia, see
tea tree
melissa, 24, 39
memory, flagging, 43
menopause, 114
menstruation, 24, 43, 114
mental state, improved, 14
mental stimulant, essential
oil, 49
Mentha x piperita,
see peppermint
mercury, 12
Mesopotamia, 11, 17
mineral oil, 38
mouth ulcers, 116

mouthwash, 121
mugwort, 11
muscle(s)
aches and pains, 43, 47,
116, 118
relaxant, 47
tension, **56**
torn, 54
myrrh, 10, 16, 18, 30, 37,
48, 114-17
tincture of, 121

N

neck massage, 58, 66-7,
90-6
neroli (orange blossom), 16,
18, 23, 31, 37, 39, 42, 45,
48-9, 106, 114-18, 123-5
nervous system, central,
19, 21-2
tension, chronic, 24

O

Ocymum basilicum, see
basil
oil, kinds of, 36, 38, 119
oils, essential (*see also*
individual names of)
'absolute', 17
anti-bacterial action, 19
anti-depressant, 49
aphrodisiac, 49
aromas of, 38
balancing, 19, 48
base, **36**
beneficial effect of, 22
blending, therapeutic
and aesthetic, 6, 19,
113-123
buying, **23**
chemistry of, **19-20**
description of **16-17**
extracting, **17-18**
labelling, 36
massage, **36**, **38-9**, **54**,
118, 124
medicinal, 37
mental stimulant, 49
natural versus
synthetic, **23**
normalizing, 19
organically produced,
18
perfume notes of, **48-9**
relaxing, 19, 48
properties of essential
oils, 7, **18-19**, **24-34**
scientific advance of,
11-12
selecting, **36**
skin sensitivity to, 24
stimulating, 19, 48
storage of, **23**
suppliers, 38
therapeutic and
aesthetic blending of,
113-123
thirty most commonly

used, **24-34**
undiluted, **44**
what they are, **16-17**
olfactory centre, 20-21
olive, 36, 38, 119
orange, 13, 17, 31, 37, 45-6, 106, 114-17, 119, 123-4
orange blossom *see* neroli
orange flower water, 17,
120-3
orange tree, 16
Origanum majorana, see
marjoram

P

pain, reducing, 43
patchouli, 19, 23, 31, 36-7,
42, 46, 48-9, 114-17, 119,
123-4
Pelargonium
odoratissimum, see
geranium
pepper, black, 19, 25, 37,
39, 48-9, 114-17, 124-5
peppermint, 19, 24, 32, 39,
43-5, 48-9, 107, 114-17,
121, 125
percussion *see* tapotement
perfume(s), 50, **123-5**
Arabian, 11
perfume-making
procedure, 50
notes of essential oils,
48-9
skin, **45**
synthetic, 22
perspiration, 43
petitgrain, 16, 32, 49, 106,
114-18, 123-4
petrissage (kneading) 55, *62*
phlebitis, 54
pigmentation, skin (*see*
skin)
pine, 16, 18, 37, 45-8, 106,
118-19
-like essences, 37
Scots (*Pinus sylvestris*),
32, 114–17
pioneers, twentieth-century, **13-14**
Piper nigrum, see pepper,
black
plant(s)
active principles of, 12
essences (*see also* oils,
essential), 10
PMS (pre-menstrual
syndrome), 114
Pogostemon patchouli, see
patchouli
Practice of Aromatherapy,
The, 13
pregnancy, 106, 107
caution, 24, 26, 28-30,
32-3, 37
pressure, massage, 110
caution, 101
massage, *101*
products, synthetic, **23**, 38

psoriasis, 105
psychiatric patients, 13
psycho-therapeutic
influences, 48
pummelling, 54, 99, *100*,
106
push-and-pull stroke, *76*

R

rashes, 54
reflexology, 78
rejuvenation, 14
reproductive system, 19
resinous essences, 37
respiratory complaints,
19, 43
restful sleep concoctions,
118
rheumatic pain, 14, 43
rheumatism, 116
riding the waves, *69*
ringworm, 116, 122
rooms, perfuming, **44-5**,
50, 125
Rosa damascena, see rose
otto
rose, 16, 18-19, 37, 46, 106
rose otto, 16, 18-19, 23, 33,
39, 42, 46, 48-9, 114-18,
123-5
rosemary *(Rosmarinus*
officinalis), 12, 18-19, 33,
37, 42-3, 45-6, 48-9, 114-17, 118-20, 123, 125
rosewater, 11, 17, 120-3
rosewood oil, 18
Rovesti, Paolo, **13**
rush, 10

S

sage, 12
Salvia sclarea, see clary
sage
sandalwood *(Santalum*
album), 11, 16, 19, 23, 33,
37, 42, 44, 46-9, 106, 114-20, 124-5
sauna, facial, **41**
scabies, 116, 122
scalds, 44
scalp massage, *97*
self-massage, **102-5**, *103*,
104, 105
sesame seed oil, 38
shoulders, **90-5**
massage, 58, *66-8*
sinusitis, 43, 116
caution, *93*
skin, 13
brushing, dry-, **105**
care, 6, **40-2**, 120-1
cells, healthy, 18
creams and
ointments, 121
oily or acneous, 38
perfumes, essential
oils as, **45**
pigmentation, 29, 31
pores, clogging of, 38

sensitive, 24, 28-9,
30-2, 34, 39, 50
tonic base, 120
smell, sense of, 6, **19**,
20-2, 50
solvents, use of, 17-18
sprains, 24, 43, 54, 114
steam inhalations (*see*
inhalations)
stings, 44, 114
stress, 7, 24
-related problems, 22,
45
striking (*see* tapotement)
stroking (*see* effleurage)
sunbathing cautions, 29-31
sunflower seed oil, 38
suppliers, essential oils 38
swellings, 43, 54

T

tapotement 54-5, **99**, 106
tea tree, 19, 34, 37, 42,
44-5, 48, 114-22
therapeutic and aesthetic
blending, **113-123**
properties of essential
oils, **24-34**
thighs massage, *72*
thyme, 19, 45
Tisserand, Robert, **14**
toothache, 43
tuberculosis, 19
tuberose, 17

U

ulcers, mouth, 116
skin, 54

V

valerian, 22
Valnet, Dr. Jean, **13**, 19
varicose veins, 54
vegetable oil, 119
vetiver *(Vetiveria*
zizanioides), 16, 34, 36-7,
42, 46, 48-9,
114-17, 119, 124-5
viral, properties, anti-,
19, 45
vitamins A and E, 38

W

witch hazel, 120
wounds, 44
cuts and grazes, 114
soldiers', 19

Y

ylang-ylang, 18-19, 24,
34, 37, 39, 42, 46-9, 106,
114-17, 119, 123-5

Z

Zingiber officinale, see
ginger